Management of Esophageal Cancer

Editors

JOHN A. FEDERICO
THOMAS FABIAN

SURGICAL CLINICS
OF NORTH AMERICA

www.surgical.theclinics.com

Consulting Editor
RONALD F. MARTIN

June 2021 • Volume 101 • Number 3

ELSEVIER

1600 John F. Kennedy Boulevard • Suite 1800 • Philadelphia, Pennsylvania, 19103-2899

http://www.surgical.theclinics.com

SURGICAL CLINICS OF NORTH AMERICA Volume 101, Number 3
June 2021 ISSN 0039–6109, ISBN-13: 978-0-323-79069-7

Editor: John Vassallo, j.vassallo@elsevier.com
Developmental Editor: Arlene Campos

Surgical Clinics of North America (ISSN 0039–6109) is published bimonthly by Elsevier Inc., 360 Park Avenue South, New York, NY 10010-1710. Months of publication are February, April, June, August, October, and December. Business and Editorial Offices: 1600 John F. Kennedy Blvd., Suite 1800, Philadelphia, PA 19103-2899. Periodicals postage paid at New York, NY and additional mailing offices. Subscription prices are $443.00 per year for US individuals, $1198.00 per year for US institutions, $100.00 per year for US & Canadian students and residents, $547.00 per year for Canadian individuals, $1270.00 per year for Canadian institutions, $536.00 for international individuals, $1270.00 per year for international institutions and $250.00 per year for foreign students/residents. To receive student/resident rate, orders must be accompanied by name of affiliated institution, date of term, and the *signature* of program/residency coordinator on institution letterhead. Orders will be billed at individual rate until proof of status is received. Foreign air speed delivery is included in all *Clinics* subscription prices. All prices are subject to change without notice. POSTMASTER: Send address changes to *Surgical Clinics*, Elsevier Health Sciences Division, Subscription Customer Service, 3251 Riverport Lane, Maryland Heights, MO 63043. **Customer Service (orders, claims, online, change of address): Telephone: 1-800-654-2452 (U.S. and Canada); 314-447-8871 (outside U.S. and Canada). Fax: 314-447-8029. E-mail: journalscustomerservice-usa@elsevier.com (for print support); journalsonlinesupport-usa@elsevier.com (for online support).**

Reprints. For copies of 100 or more, of articles in this publication, please contact the Commercial Reprints Department, Elsevier Inc., 360 Park Avenue South, New York, New York 10010-1710. Tel. 212-633-3874, Fax: 212-633-3820, E-mail: reprints@elsevier.com.

The *Surgical Clinics of North America* is also published in Spanish by McGraw-Hill Interamericana Editores S.A., P.O. Box 5-237 06500 Mexico D.F. Mexico; and in Portuguese by Interlivros Edicoes Ltda., Rua Comandante Coelho 1085, CEP 21250, Rio de Janeiro, Brazil; and in Greek by Paschalidis Medical Publications, Athens Greece.

The *Surgical Clinics of North America* is covered in *MEDLINE/PubMed (Index Medicus)*, *EMBASE/Excerpta Medica*, *Current Contents/Clinical Medicine*, *Current Contents/Life Sciences*, *Science Citation Index*, and *ISI/BIOMED*.

Contributors

CONSULTING EDITOR

RONALD F. MARTIN, MD, FACS
Colonel (Retired), United States Army Reserve, Department of General Surgery and
Surgical Oncology, Madigan Army Medical Center, Tacoma, Washington

EDITORS

JOHN A. FEDERICO, MD, FRCSC, FACS
Attending Thoracic Surgeon, Surgery, Kalispell Regional Medical Center, Kalispell
Regional Healthcare, Kalispell, Montana

THOMAS FABIAN, MD, FCCP
Chief, Section of Thoracic Surgery, Tenured Professor of Surgery and Endowed Professor
of the Catherine Sheer Britton Chair, Albany Medical College, Albany Medical Center,
Albany, New York

AUTHORS

ABBAS E. ABBAS, MD, MS, FACS
Professor and Vice Chair of Thoracic Medicine and Surgery, Department of Thoracic
Medicine and Surgery, Lewis Katz School of Medicine at Temple University; Thoracic
Surgeon-in-Chief, Temple University Health System, Philadelphia, Pennsylvania

GHULAM ABBAS, MD, MHCM, FACS
Professor and Chief, Division of Thoracic Surgery, Department of Cardiovascular and
Thoracic Surgery, Surgical Director, Thoracic Oncology WVU Cancer Institute, West
Virginia University School of Medicine, Morgantown, West Virginia

EDWIN ACEVEDO Jr. MD, MHA
General Surgery Resident, Department of Surgery, Temple University Hospital,
Philadelphia, Pennsylvania

CHARLES T. BAKHOS, MD, MS, FACS
Associate Professor, Department of Thoracic Medicine and Surgery, Division of Thoracic
Surgery, Lewis Katz School of Medicine, Temple University, Temple University Hospital,
Fox Chase Comprehensive Cancer Center, Philadelphia, Pennsylvania

ERNEST G. CHAN, MD, MPH
Resident Physician, Department of Cardiothoracic Surgery, University of Pittsburgh
School of Medicine, University of Pittsburgh Medical Center, Pittsburgh, Pennsylvania

CHIGOZIRIM N. EKEKE, MD
Resident Physician, Department of Cardiothoracic Surgery, University of Pittsburgh
School of Medicine, University of Pittsburgh Medical Center, Pittsburgh, Pennsylvania

THOMAS FABIAN, MD, FCCP
Attending Thoracic Surgeon, Chief, Section of Thoracic Surgery, Tenured Professor of Surgery and Endowed Professor of the Catherine Sheer Britton Chair, Albany Medical College, Albany Medical Center, Albany, New York

ROMULO FAJARDO, MD
General Surgery Resident, Department of Surgery, Temple University Hospital, Philadelphia, Pennsylvania

JOHN A. FEDERICO, MD, FRCSC, FACS
Attending Thoracic Surgeon, Surgery, Kalispell Regional Medical Center, Kalispell Regional Healthcare, Kalispell, Montana

EKATERINA FEDOROVA, MD
Resident Physician, Department of Surgery, MedStar Franklin Square Medical Center, Baltimore, Maryland

ROBERT HERRON, DO
Assistant Professor, Division of Thoracic Surgery, Department of Cardiovascular Surgery and Thoracic Surgery, West Virginia University, West Virginia University School of Medicine, Morgantown, West Virginia

FACUNDO IRIARTE, MD
Division of Thoracic Surgery, Department of Thoracic Medicine and Surgery, Temple University Hospital, Fox Chase Comprehensive Cancer Center, Philadelphia, Pennsylvania

MICHAEL S. KENT, MD
Division of Thoracic Surgery and Interventional Pulmonology, Department of Surgery, Beth Israel Deaconess Medical Center, Harvard Medical School, Boston, Massachusetts

ALEXANDER LEUNG, MD
Division of Cardiothoracic Surgery, Albany Medical Center, Albany, New York

JAMES D. LUKETICH, MD
Chair, Department of Cardiothoracic Surgery, University of Pittsburgh School of Medicine, University of Pittsburgh Medical Center, Pittsburgh, Pennsylvania

M. BLAIR MARSHALL, MD
Attending Surgeon, Division of Thoracic Surgery, Brigham and Women's Hospital, Boston, Massachusetts; Attending Surgeon, Division of Thoracic Surgery, West Roxbury Veterans Hospital Administration

JEREMIAH T. MARTIN, MBBCh, MSCRD, FRCSI
Senior Medical Director, Thoracic Surgery, Southern Ohio Medical Center, Portsmouth, Ohio

ROMAN V. PETROV, MD, PhD, FACS
Associate Professor, Department of Thoracic Medicine and Surgery, Division of Thoracic Surgery, Lewis Katz School of Medicine, Temple University, Temple University Hospital, Fox Chase Comprehensive Cancer Center, Philadelphia, Pennsylvania

EALAF SHEMMERI, MD
Section of Thoracic Surgery, Department of Surgery, Albany Medical College, Albany, New York

STACEY SU, MD
Division of Thoracic Surgery, Department of Thoracic Medicine and Surgery, Temple University Hospital, Fox Chase Comprehensive Cancer Center, Philadelphia, Pennsylvania

MANUEL VILLA-SANCHEZ, MD
Assistant Professor, Department of Cardiothoracic Surgery, University of Pittsburgh School of Medicine, University of Pittsburgh Medical Center, Pittsburgh, Pennsylvania

SUE XUE WANG, MD
Resident, Division of Thoracic Surgery, Brigham and Women's Hospital, Boston, Massachusetts

AMMARA A. WATKINS, MD, MPH
Division of Thoracic Surgery and Interventional Pulmonology, Department of Surgery, Beth Israel Deaconess Medical Center, Harvard Medical School, Boston, Massachusetts

THOMAS J. WATSON, MD, FACS
Professor of Surgery, Georgetown University School of Medicine, Chair of Surgery and Chief of Thoracic Surgery, MedStar Health, Washington, DC

JESSICA A. ZERILLO, MD, MPH
Division of Medical Oncology, Department of Medicine, Beth Israel Deaconess Medical Center, Harvard Medical School, Boston, Massachusetts

Contents

To care and treat patients with esophageal cancer, one must first understand the epidemiology of Barrett's esophagus (BE). BE is defined as the intestinal metaplasia occurring within the esophagus from normal squamous epithelium to abnormal specialized columnar epithelium. BE, while first described by Allison in 1948, was attributed to Norman Barrett in 1950, who reported a case of chronic peptic ulcer in the lower esophagus that was covered by columnar epithelium.

The incidence of esophageal adenocarcinoma (EAC) has risen in the United States and western Europe for over 40 years. Barrett's esophagus (BE), defined as intestinal metaplasia of the esophageal mucosa, is the precursor to EAC. As both the development and progression of BE are related to gastroesophageal reflux disease (GERD), therapies for control of GERD are important to prevent neoplastic progression in susceptible individuals. Endoscopic resective and ablative techniques have been popularized in recent years to eliminate pathologic esophageal mucosa in early stages. Utilizing these approaches, EAC can be prevented or cured prior to the development of advanced esophageal malignancy with its lethal consequences.

Optimal treatment of esophageal cancer is a complex process dependent on many factors, including stage at diagnosis, medical fitness, physician judgment, and expertise. Despite significant advances in understanding of this cancer, survival remains low. Identifying patients with early-stage disease can enhance their outcomes dramatically. On a broader scale, staging is critical in advancing the quality of care delivered to these patients now and in the future. This article is designed to review clinicians' expertise with staging and to elaborate on the nuances frequently encountered when doing so.

With advancing endoscopic technology and screening protocols for Barrett's disease, more patients are being diagnosed with early-stage esophageal cancer. These early-stage patients may be amendable to endoscopic therapies, such as endomucosal resection and ablation. These therapies may minimize morbidity, but the elevated risk of recurrence cannot be overlooked. This article reports outcomes and recommendations for surveillance and management of recurrent esophageal cancer following endoscopic therapies.

 Video content accompanies this article at http://www.surgical.theclinics.com.

Esophageal cancer is the eighth most common cancer worldwide, and its incidence has been increasing over the past several decades. Esophagectomy currently is the standard of care for more advanced early esophageal cancer and should be performed at centers of excellence with high volumes, appropriate supportive staff, and multidisciplinary expertise.

Definitive chemoradiation therapy avoids the perioperative and long-term morbidity of esophagectomy and is the standard of care for cervical esophageal cancer. There are significant differences in tumor response to chemoradiation and recurrence patterns between squamous cell cancer and adenocarcinoma of the esophagus. Multimodality therapy for esophageal cancer continues to progress, now with the widespread use of PET scanning and possible active surveillance in patients with complete clinical response to chemoradiation. As drug development and targeted therapy trials continue to expand, our understanding of tumor biology and precision medicine will continue to refine the treatment of esophageal cancer.

Trimodality therapy, or the use of concurrent chemoradiation followed by surgery, is the cornerstone of contemporary management of esophageal cancer. This article discusses the landmark trials and most current data to understand the concepts, applications, and outcomes from trimodality therapy in locally advanced esophageal cancer.

multiple techniques, as occasionally the clinical situation may be better suited for a particular technique. Regardless of the method of creating the esophagogastric anastomosis, the goal is to create a viable, tension-free and nonobstructive anastomosis with adequate margins.

 Video content accompanies this article at http://www.surgical. theclinics.com.

Newer surgical techniques have reduced complications and mortality following esophagectomy, but they nevertheless remain high. Data regarding complications are frequently inconsistent and, therefore, difficult to compare between groups. As a result, considerable energy is spent trying to identify best practices to minimize complications. This article reviews the rates of complications and attempts to give guidance regarding their management and outcomes.

SURGICAL CLINICS OF NORTH AMERICA

SERIES OF RELATED INTEREST

Advances in Surgery
https://www.advancessurgery.com/
Surgical Oncology Clinics
https://www.surgonc.theclinics.com/
Thoracic Surgery Clinics
http://www.thoracic.theclinics.com/

THE CLINICS ARE AVAILABLE ONLINE!
Access your subscription at:
www.theclinics.com

Foreword

Esophageal Surgery

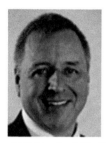

Ronald F. Martin, MD, FACS
Consulting Editor

There are some clinical interests and perhaps even some organs that don't fit neatly into one recognized discipline. These clinical entities either seemed to have multiple parents or are orphans—frequently depending on what problem has developed or, more likely, when the problem develops (such as nights or weekends). The world of clinical concerns related to the esophagus appears to me to be a prime illustrator of this concept. Depending on the situation, thoracic surgeons, general surgeons, gastro-enterologists, otolaryngologists, minimally invasive surgeons, surgical oncologists, foregut surgeons, and probably a few other specialties I have left out, all lay claim to the esophageal dominion. On some occasions, many of them rapidly point to a specialty other than their own when problems arise. Overall, both concepts make some sense in varying situations.

As the readers of this series may recall, we have wrestled with tensions of what should best be served by the generalist and what may better be tackled by the specialist. And, readers of this series may also recall that there has frequently been no one right answer to that question. Often, it is local factors and reality that trump broad theory when addressing this concern. The esophagus presents us with a somewhat rare variation to this conundrum in that it begs us to find the unusual person who is a generalized specialist or a specialized generalist.

As Drs Federico and Fabian along with their colleagues describe in this issue of the *Surgical Clinics*, there is a need for all of the skill sets of the specialties listed above (along with a whole host of other specialty input: diagnostic imaging and interventional radiology, medical oncology, radiation oncology, nutritional support, intensive care [medical or surgical], pulmonology, palliative care, and so on) to take care of patients with esophageal disorders. On a systems level, all of these disciplines are needed and valued. However, when situations deteriorate and we have a patient who has developed a tracheoesophageal fistula, esophageal perforation, obstruction, or hemorrhage, then perhaps we may need to narrow the team a bit.

Surg Clin N Am 101 (2021) xiii–xv
https://doi.org/10.1016/j.suc.2021.04.001
0039-6109/21/© 2021 Published by Elsevier Inc.

One general administrative principle is that it is rarely a good idea to be "one-deep" on the bench for any medical discipline. It is even worse to be "one-deep" for a medical discipline that responds to life-threatening emergencies. That accepted, it is a challenge for all but a very few centers to have enough volume of patients to have significant depth on their esophageal bench in multiple disciplines. We must therefore balance how much we concentrate the skill sets required into any given service or individual. This balancing act between individuals and services can at times be challenging. It must be done though because, despite our best efforts, there is a limit to how many problems we can solve with waiting for help to arrive or transferring patients long distances.

Having someone who can comfortably operate in the chest, neck, and abdomen as well as perform diagnostic and therapeutic endoscopy is a huge boon to any clinical staff. That kind of capability may not always be available 24/7 at many institutions. In such circumstances, it may fall upon an individual or multiple people with some of these skills to have to step up in difficult times. Under such circumstances, the goal will often be to temporize the situation adequately to allow the patient to be united with a team that has greater clinical capacity.

The information presented in this issue will help any clinician better familiarize herself or himself with the issues that matter for patients with esophageal disorders of a wide variety. As important as this information will be to help you make the correct first step, it may be just as important to help you prevent making an incorrect first step. The care of the patient with an esophageal malady can be extremely rewarding, but it is often even more extremely unforgiving.

If you will permit me to add some unsolicited advice, in our age of "nondirect" communication (texting, e-mail, and so forth), I would encourage anyone who encounters patients with serious esophageal pathologic condition and wishes advice to call directly and speak one-on-one to someone with expertise on the subject. The cadre of people who do this sort of work with great routine is small and scattered about, yet I have found that they all seem to have phones and generally tend to answer them promptly. Sometimes a 5-minute conversation can save hours of misery later, not to mention benefit the patient.

We are indebted to the efforts of Dr Federico, Dr Fabian, and their colleagues for assembling this excellent collection of articles. They have answered our calls and have been extremely generous in sharing their time and thoughts on a topic that they all hold very dear. I owe an extra personal debt to Dr Federico in that he has been a mentor and role model to me since my days in medical school. I have learned much from him both directly and indirectly for many decades. Possibly one of the most important lessons learned is to reinforce how much we all need each other to turn to when we need advice on just about anything. A career in surgery can last a long time.

We all need friends and mentors who can help us when we need guidance and guide us when we may not think we need help.

Ronald F. Martin, MD, FACS
Colonel (retired), United States Army Reserve
Department of General Surgery and
Surgical Oncology
Madigan Army Medical Center
9040 Jackson Avenue
Tacoma, WA 98431, USA

E-mail address:
rfmcescna@gmail.com

Preface

Surgical Family

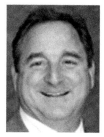 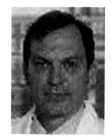

John A. Federico, MD   Thomas Fabian, MD, FCCP
Editors

It was an honor to participate in the creation of this issue. Thoracic Surgeons have the privilege of being a small tightknit surgical family. Smaller yet is the field of esophageal surgery. In the care of these patients, esophageal cancer has tamed our egos as a consequence of an unforgiving organ.

Assisting with the production of this issue of *Surgical Clinics* has given me the opportunity to reflect on a 30-year career in thoracic surgery. It brings to light the names of those who have come before me and who passed their knowledge onto me, and to those whom I have helped train (for better or worse), and who continue to train the next generation. Choosing our article authors, we paid specific attention to diverse ideas and perspectives, honoring those who have contributed significantly to the field. It has been a wonderful experience working so closely with the authors and in doing so I have learned so much.

Ronald Belsey, MD and Griff Pearson, MD, both of whom had a role in my training at the latter term of their professional careers, refer to esophageal surgery as a relative "no man's land" in the field of surgery. The esophagus is an unforgiving organ and not an ideal proving ground for the "occasional operator." Only a select committed group can accomplish truly great outcomes. As Belsey was fond of saying in regards to esophageal cancer, others "took it up, mucked it up, and then gave it up."

The authors of this *Surgical Clinics* are part of a family of surgeons who have confronted this unforgiving organ, not as an occasional undertaking, but as a frontier from which to learn and improve upon. Many of the authors in this issue have learned from each other at formal training programs, at professional meetings, or as partners. We readily share our knowledge, experience, and biases or foibles within these articles. We are a small family, always ready to learn, to teach, to improve for the sake of patients.

Surg Clin N Am 101 (2021) xvii–xviii
https://doi.org/10.1016/j.suc.2021.03.014
0039-6109/21/© 2021 Published by Elsevier Inc.

surgical.theclinics.com

It is our hope that this *Surgical Clinics*, and articles herein, will help some of you to advance the field of esophageal surgery and improve the outcomes of our patients with esophageal cancer.

John A. Federico, MD, FRCSC
Chief of Thoracic Surgery, Kalispell Regional Medical Center
Kalispell Regional Healthcare Surgical Specialists
1333 Surgical Services Drive
Kalispell, MT 59901, USA

Thomas Fabian, MD, FCCP
Thoracic Surgery, Albany Medical College
50 New Scotland Avenue, Third Floor
Albany, NY 12159, USA

E-mail addresses:
jfederico@krmc.org (J.A. Federico)
Fabiant@amc.edu (T. Fabian)

Dedication

"To both of our families, especially to our children, who ultimately sacrifice time with their fathers so we can care for others.
   We love you, Angela, Andrew, Tyler, Brianna, Drew, and Dixie."

John A. Federico
Thomas Fabian

Surg Clin N Am 101 (2021) xix
https://doi.org/10.1016/j.suc.2021.05.001
0039-6109/21/© 2021 Published by Elsevier Inc.

Epidemiology of Barrett's Esophagus and Esophageal Carcinoma

Thomas Fabian*, Alexander Leung

KEYWORDS

- Esophageal cancer • Barrett's esophagus • Esophageal dysplasia
- High-grade dysplasia • Low-grade dysplasia • Epidemiology

INTRODUCTION

Barrett's esophagus (BE) is typically categorized by the length or extent of metaplasia and secondly by cellular changes in the columnar epithelium.[1,2] The length of extent of metaplasia is referred to as long segment, if greater than 3 cm, and short segment, if less than 3 cm. Cellular changes refer to the metaplastic changes in the esophageal lining, changing from normal squamous to columnar epithelium; dysplasia (presence of abnormal cells) may be present or absent within the columnar epithelium. When absent, it is simply called BE; when dysplasia is present, it is referred to as low-grade dysplasia (LGD) or high-grade dysplasia (HGD). BE represents the single largest risk for the development of esophageal adenocarcinoma (EAC).

EPIDEMIOLOGY OF BARRETT'S ESOPHAGUS

BE is a relatively common condition occurring when normal squamous epithelium within the esophagus changes to columnar epithelium. The overall prevalence of the disease is difficult to define and can be seen in up to 15% of otherwise well patients suffering from gastroesophageal reflux disease (GERD).[3] Freitas and colleagues[4] reported rates in patients without GERD to be slightly lower, 8% in men and 4% in women. In 961 patients undergoing endoscopy at a large center, 6.8% were found to have BE[5]; the number was higher in patients with heartburn (8.3%) compared with those without heartburn (5.6%). Not surprisingly, the incidence of BE climbs as a result of increasing health care access and increased utilization of upper endoscopy. However, access to health care varies with socioeconomic status, which results in difficulties identifying the true prevalence of this disease.

Caucasian men in their sixth and seventh decades of life are most likely to develop BE but variations are frequent. Men are much more likely than women to have BE with ratios of 2:1 or 3:1,[4] and older patients are more likely than younger ones to have BE. Also, when comparing men and women with BE, men generally develop BE 20 years

* Corresponding author.
E-mail address: Fabiant@amc.edu

Surg Clin N Am 101 (2021) 381–389
https://doi.org/10.1016/j.suc.2021.03.001
surgical.theclinics.com
0039-6109/21/© 2021 Elsevier Inc. All rights reserved.

earlier than women.[6] The incidence of BE is highest in the Caucasian population and is 4 times more common than in African Americans.[7]

Risks factors for the development of BE include genetic factors but also include environmental exposure and patient clinical risks. Studies have shown multiple environmental factors to increase the risk of BE. Smoking of tobacco products significantly increases risk of development of BE. Cook and colleagues[8] published a meta-analysis in 2012 demonstrating progression of risk at different exposure points. Patients who smoked were significantly more likely than nonsmokers to develop BE, and increased pack years was associated with greater risk. Cook in the same paper also demonstrated that patients who smoked and had GERD had a higher risk of developing cancer compared with those who smoked and did not have GERD. The investigators suggested a synergistic effect between the two. Although epidemiologic studies vary, it is generally accepted that smoking is an independent risk factor for the development of esophageal cancer. Smokeless tobacco, specifically chewing tobacco, is a known risk factor for esophageal cancer and is widely considered a risk for squamous cell cancer (SCC) of the esophagus, and it likely is a risk of developing EAC as well.[9]

Interestingly, alcohol is not considered a risk for development of BE, although it has a strong relationship with the development of SCC, which is discuss later. Likewise, Helicobacter pylori is a risk for gastric cancer including gastroesophageal junction (GEJ) adenocarcinomas but it does not seem to be a risk for the development of BE.[10]

Patient risk factors for BE include obesity, GERD, and hiatal hernia. Obesity remains a growing problem in the developed world and is an independent risk factor for the development of BE. In a meta-analysis in 2009, Kamat and colleagues[11] showed that obese patients with a body mass index (BMI) greater than 30 were more likely to develop BE although there are articles that argue against this causation.[12] As a surrogate to BMI, others have looked at central obesity, and still others have looked at waist circumference. Kubo and colleagues[13] used waist circumference and found that men and women with increased waist circumference were at increased risk of BE and that women were at a higher risk with increased waist circumference when compared with men. BMI may be skewed by variations in muscle mass; however, central or truncal obesity may better represent the role of weight and obesity on BE.

Hiatal hernia has a clear association with BE and GERD. Although some patients may be asymptomatic, many of those patients suffer from silent reflux when measured objectively. GERD remains one of the greatest risk factors for developing BE as described earlier. Risk factors that predispose patients with GERD to BE include symptom severity, age of symptoms, and duration of symptoms.[14] It should be stated that reflux symptoms themselves are not always corroborated by objectively measured acid reflux. Andrici and colleagues[15] in their meta-analysis associated the presence of a hiatal hernia with an increased risk of BE. They also showed that a hiatal hernia was strongly associated with long-segment BE. Although most patients with BE have hiatal hernias, it has been shown that these patients generally had longer hernias and wider hiatal openings.[16]

Mitigation of risks for BE as well as risks of progression to EAC are discussed in the next chapter in this textbook.

Table 1 demonstrates commonly accepted risk and nonrisk factors for the development of BE.

EPIDEMIOLOGY OF ESOPHAGEAL CANCER

Esophageal cancers occur anywhere within the esophagus. It is generally accepted that these cancers include tumors from the cricopharyngeal muscle to the GEJ.

Table 1 Risk of Barrett's esophagus		
Patient Demographics	**Patient Risk Factors**	**Nonrisk Factors**
Male	GERD	Alcohol consumption
White	Smoking	*H pylori*
6th–7th decade	Central obesity	
	Waist circumference	
	Hiatal hernia	

Although most malignant tumors originate from the mucosa, they can originate from any layer of the esophagus. Presently, and for the last 30 years, adenocarcinomas are the most common cancer of the esophagus in North America, followed by squamous cell carcinomas of the esophagus, which typically occur in the first and second portion of the esophagus although they can occur in the third portion of the esophagus as well. Other malignancies occur in the esophagus, including small cell carcinoma, melanomas, carcinosarcoma, and gastrointestinal stromal tumors, but represent less than 1% each. This article focuses on the most common tumors seen.

According to the National Cancer Institute's Surveillance, Epidemiology, and End Results Program (SEER) Program, 17,650 esophageal cancers were diagnosed in the United States in 2019.[3] This number represented approximately 1.0% of all new cancer cases and is the 18th most common cancer in the United States. The 5-year survival was 19.9% (between 2009 and2015) and estimated deaths in 2019 were 16,080. Despite the change and increasing frequency frequently reported in literature according to SEER database, prevalence and death rates have remained fairly consistent over the last 20 years.

Lifetime risk of developing esophageal cancer is approximately 0.5% in the United States based on SEER data. The annual incidence of esophageal cancer is approximately 4.3/100,000 persons. It occurs more frequently in men (7.3) than women (1.7) per 100,000 individuals. Incidence per 100,000 is 7.8 and 6.1 in Caucasians and black men respectively and 1.8 and 2.0 in Caucasian and black women respectively. Median age of diagnosis is 68 years and 79.7% of patients fall between the age of 55 and 84 years.

At the time of diagnosis, most of the esophageal cancers are fairly advanced. With surveillance of BE, early tumors are found but for patients presenting with dysphagia, the clinical stage at diagnosis is frequently advanced. SEER data from 1998 to 2009 showed that the 35% of patients have metastasized at time of diagnosis, 30% have regional spread to lymph nodes, 22% have localized disease confined to the esophagus, and 13% are unknown stage.[17] This advanced stage at the time of diagnosis is a major contributor to the poor 5-year survival. Survival in the SEER database between 2009 and 2015 is 19.9%, which was 16,080 deaths in 2019 and a total of 2.6% of all deaths from malignancy. SCC of the esophagus was typically diagnosed at an earlier stage than EAC.[3] Esophageal cancers were treated with chemotherapy in 61.7% of patients, with radiotherapy in 55.4% of patients, and with surgery in only 26.6% of patients.[3] Patients with adenocarcinoma were twice as likely to undergo esophagectomy (32.9% vs 15.9%) compared with patients with SCCs.[3] Trimodality treatment was used in 17.8% of patients with EAC and 8.4% with SCC.

ESOPHAGEAL ADENOCARCINOMA

Although the incidence of squamous cell tumors has dropped, this decline has been made up for by an increase in EACs. EAC is most common in Caucasian men and a male-to-female ratio approaches 8:1.[18] According to SEER data, EAC seems to occur in Caucasian to African Americans at a ratio of approximately 5:1. This ratio mirrors the prevalence of BE as described earlier in this article. Risk factors for EAC are different than that of SCC and are listed on **Table 2**. Some notable differences are GERD, BE, obesity, and alcohol.

The relationship of GERD to EAC is undeniable. Not only is the presence of GERD a risk factor for BE, it is a precursor for esophageal cancer; the severity of symptoms and duration of symptoms further increase the risk of development.[19] BE is an enormous risk factor for development of EAC, and a section of this article is dedicated to that topic. Obesity is a risk factor not only for the development of BE but also for the development of EAC. In a prospective study by Abnet and colleagues,[20] obesity was shown to be a significant risk factor and is further increased with patients with higher BMI.[20] Smokers have a higher risk of developing esophageal cancer, and, at least in some studies, risk was further increased by dose of exposure.[21] In the same study, Cook and colleagues also demonstrated that patients who smoked and had GERD had a higher risk of developing cancer compared with those who smoked and did not have GERD. Although epidemiologic studies vary, it is generally accepted that smoking is an independent risk factor for the development of esophageal cancer and that its cessation is associated with reduced risk of EAC.[21]

Alcohol surprisingly does not contribute to the development of EAC. Alcohol remains a huge risk factor for SCC but not for EAC. In multiple studies, the degree of alcohol consumption and the duration of consumption were not associated with increased risk for EAC.[22] Alcohol is a risk factor for the development of gastric cancer. This observation demonstrates the difference between EAC and gastric cancer and leaves GEJ adenocarcinoma poorly defined.

H pylori is associated with development of gastric cancer but not EAC. In a large meta-analysis, H pylori has been associated with a decreased risk of 39% to 64% of BE and 52% reduction of EAC.[23] This inverse association is not well understood, although some consider gastric atrophy secondary to H pylori infection to result in reduced acid production.[18] In particular, the cagA + strain has been inversely

Table 2
Risks for malignancy of the esophagus

Histologic Type	Barrett's Esophagus	Adenocarcinoma	Squamous Cell Carcinoma	Gastric Cancer
Barrett's esophagus	−	+	−	U/I
Hiatal hernia	+	+	−	−
Smoking	+	+	+	+
Central obesity	+	+		+
H pylori	−	−	−	+
Smokeless Tobacco	−	U/I	+	U/I
ETOH	−	−	+	+
HPV	−	−	+	U/I
Proton Pump Inhibitors	−	−	−	−

Abbreviation: U/I, unknown, insufficient evidence.

associated with BE and EAC. Doorakers and colleagues[10] performed a large study looking to see if eradication of *H pylori* increased the risk of malignancy and found no evidence to suggest that.

The common perception of clinicians and lay people is that medications that result in the reduction of acid reduces risk of BE and EAC. There is little or no evidence to support this misconception, suggesting the real risk of BE and EAC is reflux alone regardless of the acid state. Data on surgical reflux control are limited as well. In a meta-analysis from 2016, antireflux surgery may prevent EAC better than medical therapy; however, antireflux surgery alone does not seem to reduce the progression to EAC back to the baseline cancer risk.[24] In addition, antireflux surgery may decrease, but not eliminate, the progression of BE to dysplasia.[25,26] It was noted that patients who had short-segment BE tended to show more regression than those with long-segment BE.

ESOPHAGEAL SQUAMOUS CELL

SCC of the esophagus typically occurs in the proximal two-thirds of the esophagus but can occur anywhere in the esophagus. According to the SEER database, the incidence of SCC in the United States continues to drop and is presently at an all-time low. Internationally, however, squamous cell carcinoma of the esophagus remains the predominate malignancy of the esophagus worldwide at approximately 90% of all cases.[27] The decreases seen in the United States may be related to decreasing rates of tobacco use.[28] This trend is consistent with reduction of total risk of esophageal cancer as duration of smoking cessation increases.[21]

The predominate risk factors for development of SCC are smoking, tobacco, alcohol, and diet and have been well-documented in the literature.[27] Human papillomavirus, which is a viral instigator of many SCCs, has been shown to increase the risk of esophageal SCC[29]; however, other studies have shown that its clinical relevance may be overstated in regard to esophageal cancer.[30] Overall, African Americans in the United States are considered at an increased risk[3] compared with the Caucasian population. According to SEER data, African Americans accounted for only 2.7% of EAC; conversely, they accounted for 26.22% of SCC.

PROGRESSION FROM BARRETT'S ESOPHAGUS

As alluded earlier in the article, BE is a precursor to the development of EAC. The diagnosis of BE is traditionally made endoscopically. On histology, the presence of specialized columnar epithelium with mucin-containing goblet cells on biopsy is diagnostic of BE.[31] In addition, the Prague classification has been used to help clinicians define the grade of Barrett's segment based on the circumferential length and maximal length.[32]

Prague C&M Criteria
  Based on endoscopic suspicion of BE:
  Measurements are made for the proximal margin of circumferential length of BE and the proximal margin for longest "tongue-like" segment of BE
  C—length from most proximal margin of circumferential BE to GEJ
  M—length from most proximal margin of longest "tongue-like" segment of BE to GEJ

The progression from BE to EAC is a spectrum that spans from LGD to HGD to ultimately EAC. The predictability of this progression and the desire to detect the disease earlier in the progression has led to the Seattle biopsy protocol[33] to identify patients with

Table 3 Annual incidence of progression of Barrett's dysplasia		
Barrett's Esophagus	**Low-Grade Dysplasia**	**High-Grade Dysplasia**
→LGD 3.6%/y	→HGD 1.19%/y	→EAC 6.6%/y
→HGD 0.78%/y	→EAC 0.54%/y	
→EAC 0.12%/y		

HGD or EAC. This protocol consists of 4 quadrant biopsies every 1 to 2 cm in areas of mucosal abnormalities. The testing interval depends on the histologic findings of the biopsy. For patients with no dysplasia, the recommended surveillance interval is 3 years. However, once the low-grade dysplasia is detected, annual endoscopy is recommended. Patients who have HGD either undergo invasive therapies or require endoscopy every 3 months. Other adjuncts to aid in detecting progression include using chromoendoscopy, narrow-band imaging, and autofluorescence endoscopy.

Recommended Surveillance Interval	Years
No dysplasia	3 y
LGD	1 y
HGD	3 mo

Because it is known that not all patients with BE will progress to EAC,[34] it is important to attempt to identify risk factors in this specific patient group. Other papers have described risk factors of progression: age, male sex, white race, central obesity, smoking, family history of BE or EAC, time duration of BE, length of Barrett's segment, and GERD.[35] These risk factors have been elucidated in prior sections and just emphasis the synergistic effect relationship between BE and EAC. One recent retrospective study confirmed the risk factors of age, obesity, and smoking as risk factors for patients with BE that were followed and ultimately progressed to HGD or EAC.[36] Interestingly, other risk factors of diabetes, caffeine, and colonic adenomas were introduced in this study. These risk factors are not difficult to understand as the diabetes and caffeine both can worsen GERD, which again is a primary risk factor for BE and EAC. The risk factor of colonic adenoma has been described previously in the literature[37] and proposes that there may be a genetic component in the progression of BE to EAC.

Lastly, the endoscopic finding of LGD or HGD seems to be one of the strongest risk factors for progression to EAC.[14,36] At first this fact may seem trivial; it suggests that the progression from BE to EAC while continuous may not be linear but may be exponential in growth. It also reemphasizes the role of early detection of dysplasia in the endoscopic evaluation algorithm. Individual risk factors aside, the incidence of progression is shown in **Table 3**.[34,38–41]

SUMMARY

BE remains the most important risk factor for the progression to EAC. Although there are many individual risk factors that are unique to each specific pathology, the clinician needs to understand that the progression from BE to EAC is a continuum with a synergistic effect of each risk factor to the ultimate development of EAC. Many of the risk factors are beyond the patient's control; however, limiting the specific patient factors (ie, obesity and smoking) can still play a role in prevention. Lastly, the symptoms of

GERD should never be dismissed as such without endoscopy, especially in the role of persistent or worsening symptoms.

REFERENCES

1. Allison PR. Peptic ulcer of the oesophagus. Thorax 1948;3(1):20–42.
2. Barrett NR. Chronic peptic ulcer of the oesophagus and 'oesophagitis'. Br J Surg 1950;38(150):175–82.
3. Then EO, Lopez M, Saleem S, et al. Esophageal Cancer: An Updated Surveillance Epidemiology and End Results Database Analysis. World J Oncol 2020; 11(2):55–64.
4. Freitas MC, Moretzsohn LD, Coelho LG. Prevalence of Barrett's esophagus in individuals without typical symptoms of gastroesophageal reflux disease. Arq Gastroenterol 2008;45(1):46–9.
5. Rex DK, Cummings OW, Shaw M, et al. Screening for Barrett's esophagus in colonoscopy patients with and without heartburn. Gastroenterology 2003;125(6): 1670–7.
6. van Blankenstein M, Looman CW, Johnston BJ, et al. Age and sex distribution of the prevalence of Barrett's esophagus found in a primary referral endoscopy center. Am J Gastroenterol 2005;100(3):568–76.
7. Alkaddour A, Palacio C, Vega KJ. Risk of histologic Barrett's esophagus between African Americans and non-Hispanic whites: A meta-analysis. United Eur Gastroenterol J 2018;6(1):22–8.
8. Cook MB, Shaheen NJ, Anderson LA, et al. Cigarette smoking increases risk of Barrett's esophagus: an analysis of the Barrett's and Esophageal Adenocarcinoma Consortium. Gastroenterology 2012;142(4):744–53.
9. Sinha DN, Abdulkader RS, Gupta PC. Smokeless tobacco-associated cancers: A systematic review and meta-analysis of Indian studies. Int J Cancer 2016;138(6): 1368–79.
10. Doorakkers E, Lagergren J, Santoni G, et al. Helicobacter pylori eradication treatment and the risk of Barrett's esophagus and esophageal adenocarcinoma. Helicobacter 2020;25(3):e12688.
11. Kamat P, Wen S, Morris J, et al. Exploring the association between elevated body mass index and Barrett's esophagus: a systematic review and meta-analysis. Ann Thorac Surg 2009;87(2):655–62.
12. Seidel D, Muangpaisan W, Hiro H, et al. The association between body mass index and Barrett's esophagus: a systematic review. Dis Esophagus 2009;22(7): 564–70.
13. Kubo A, Cook MB, Shaheen NJ, et al. Sex-specific associations between body mass index, waist circumference and the risk of Barrett's oesophagus: a pooled analysis from the international BEACON consortium. Gut 2013;62(12):1684–91.
14. Chang JT, Katzka DA. Gastroesophageal reflux disease, Barrett esophagus, and esophageal adenocarcinoma. Arch Intern Med 2004;164(14):1482–8.
15. Andrici J, Tio M, Cox MR, et al. Hiatal hernia and the risk of Barrett's esophagus. J Gastroenterol Hepatol 2013;28(3):415–31.
16. Cameron AJ. Barrett's esophagus: prevalence and size of hiatal hernia. Am J Gastroenterol 1999;94(8):2054–9.
17. Zhang Y. Epidemiology of esophageal cancer. World J Gastroenterol 2013; 19(34):5598–606.
18. Coleman HG, Xie SH, Lagergren J. The epidemiology of esophageal adenocarcinoma. Gastroenterology 2018;154(2):390–405.

19. Cook MB, Corley DA, Murray LJ, et al. Gastroesophageal reflux in relation to adenocarcinomas of the esophagus: a pooled analysis from the Barrett's and Esophageal Adenocarcinoma Consortium (BEACON). PLoS One 2014;9(7): e103508.

20. Abnet CC, Freedman ND, Hollenbeck AR, et al. A prospective study of BMI and risk of oesophageal and gastric adenocarcinoma. Eur J Cancer 2008;44(3): 465–71.

21. Cook MB, Kamangar F, Whiteman DC, et al. Cigarette smoking and adenocarcinomas of the esophagus and esophagogastric junction: a pooled analysis from the international BEACON consortium. J Natl Cancer Inst 2010;102(17):1344–53.

22. Tramacere I, Pelucchi C, Bagnardi V, et al. A meta-analysis on alcohol drinking and esophageal and gastric cardia adenocarcinoma risk. Ann Oncol 2012; 23(2):287–97.

23. Rokkas T, Pistiolas D, Sechopoulos P, et al. Relationship between Helicobacter pylori infection and esophageal neoplasia: a meta-analysis. Clin Gastroenterol Hepatol 2007;5(12):1417 e1-2.

24. Maret-Ouda J, Konings P, Lagergren J, et al. Antireflux Surgery and Risk of Esophageal Adenocarcinoma: A Systematic Review and Meta-analysis. Ann Surg 2016;263(2):251–7.

25. Allaix ME, Patti MG. Antireflux surgery for dysplastic Barrett. World J Surg 2015; 39(3):588–94.

26. Knight BC, Devitt PG, Watson DI, et al. Long-term Efficacy of Laparoscopic Antireflux Surgery on Regression of Barrett's Esophagus Using BRAVO Wireless pH Monitoring: A Prospective Clinical Cohort Study. Ann Surg 2017;266(6):1000–5.

27. Abnet CC, Arnold M, Wei WQ. Epidemiology of Esophageal Squamous Cell Carcinoma. Gastroenterology 2018;154(2):360–73.

28. Jamal A, Phillips E, Gentzke AS, et al. Current Cigarette Smoking Among Adults - United States, 2016. MMWR Morb Mortal Wkly Rep 2018;67(2):53–9.

29. Hardefeldt HA, Cox MR, Eslick GD. Association between human papillomavirus (HPV) and oesophageal squamous cell carcinoma: a meta-analysis. Epidemiol Infect 2014;142(6):1119–37.

30. Bucchi D, Stracci F, Buonora N, et al. Human papillomavirus and gastrointestinal cancer: A review. World J Gastroenterol 2016;22(33):7415–30.

31. Salemme M, Villanacci V, Cengia G, et al. Intestinal metaplasia in Barrett's oesophagus: An essential factor to predict the risk of dysplasia and cancer development. Dig Liver Dis 2016;48(2):144–7.

32. Sharma P, Dent J, Armstrong D, et al. The development and validation of an endoscopic grading system for Barrett's esophagus: the Prague C & M criteria. Gastroenterology 2006;131(5):1392–9.

33. Schoofs N, Bisschops R, Prenen H. Progression of Barrett's esophagus toward esophageal adenocarcinoma: an overview. Ann Gastroenterol 2017;30(1):1–6.

34. Hvid-Jensen F, Pedersen L, Drewes AM, et al. Incidence of adenocarcinoma among patients with Barrett's esophagus. N Engl J Med 2011;365(15):1375–83.

35. Krishnamoorthi R, Borah B, Heien H, et al. Rates and predictors of progression to esophageal carcinoma in a large population-based Barrett's esophagus cohort. Gastrointest Endosc 2016;84(1):40.e7.

36. Kambhampati S, Tieu AH, Luber B, et al. Risk Factors for Progression of Barrett's Esophagus to High Grade Dysplasia and Esophageal Adenocarcinoma. Sci Rep 2020;10(1):4899.

37. Kumaravel A, Thota PN, Lee HJ, et al. Higher prevalence of colon polyps in patients with Barrett's esophagus: a case-control study. Gastroenterol Rep (Oxf) 2014;2(4):281–7.

38. Wani S, Falk G, Hall M, et al. Patients with nondysplastic Barrett's esophagus have low risks for developing dysplasia or esophageal adenocarcinoma. Clin Gastroenterol Hepatol 2011;9(3):220.e26 [quiz: e26].

39. Yousef F, Cardwell C, Cantwell MM, et al. The incidence of esophageal cancer and high-grade dysplasia in Barrett's esophagus: a systematic review and meta-analysis. Am J Epidemiol 2008;168(3):237–49.

40. Singh S, Manickam P, Amin AV, et al. Incidence of esophageal adenocarcinoma in Barrett's esophagus with low-grade dysplasia: a systematic review and meta-analysis. Gastrointest Endosc 2014;79(6):897–909.e4 [quiz: 983.e1, 983.e3].

41. Rastogi A, Puli S, El-Serag HB, et al. Incidence of esophageal adenocarcinoma in patients with Barrett's esophagus and high-grade dysplasia: a meta-analysis. Gastrointest Endosc 2008;67(3):394–8.

Antireflux and Endoscopic Therapies for Barrett Esophagus and Superficial Esophageal Neoplasia

Ekaterina Fedorova, MD[a], Thomas J. Watson, MD[b],*

KEYWORDS

- Barrett esophagus • Esophageal adenocarcinoma
- Gastroesophageal reflux disease • Endoscopic resection • Radiofrequency ablation

KEY POINTS

- Esophageal adenocarcinoma (EAC) has been increasing in incidence for over forty years and carries a poor prognosis, largely due to its advanced stage at the time of its typical presentation and the lack of curative systemic therapies.
- To decrease mortality from EAC, efforts must be made to decrease its incidence or to detect and treat it at an early, curable stage.
- Gastroesophageal reflux disease (GERD) promotes both the development and progression of Barrett's esophagus, the precursor of EAC. Control of GERD, with either acid suppressive medications or antireflux surgery, can help prevent the development of EAC.
- Endoscopic resective and ablative techniques to treat superficial esophageal neoplasia have been popularized in recent years, largely replacing esophagectomy as the treatments of choice in appropriately selected cases of early disease.

INTRODUCTION

Esophageal carcinoma is a highly lethal malignancy with a poor prognosis. The American Cancer Society predicted 18,440 new cases of esophageal cancer in the United States (US) in 2020 with 16,170 deaths.[1] Based on data from the National Cancer Institute Surveillance, Epidemiology, and End Results 2018 registry, the 5-year relative survival from esophageal cancer in the United States between 2010 and 2016 was 19.9%.[2] Survival rates for esophageal carcinoma, however, are dependent on the stage at the time of diagnosis. Superficial esophageal neoplasia is highly curable;

Author commercial or financial conflicts: None.
Author funding sources: None.
[a] MedStar Franklin Square Medical Center, 9000 Franklin Square Drive, Department of Surgery, Baltimore, MD 21237, USA; [b] MedStar Georgetown University Hospital, 3800 Reservoir Rd, NW, 4PHC Department of Surgery, Washington, DC 20007, USA
* Corresponding author.
E-mail address: tjwmd9@gmail.com

Surg Clin N Am 101 (2021) 391–403
https://doi.org/10.1016/j.suc.2021.03.002
0039-6109/21/© 2021 Elsevier Inc. All rights reserved.
surgical.theclinics.com

the therapeutic pessimism accompanying advanced carcinoma is not appropriate in early cases. As esophageal cancer typically causes symptoms only with advanced disease, diagnosis before symptom onset yields the best chance of cure.

Although squamous cell carcinoma represents 90% of all esophageal cancer worldwide, and was the predominant histologic subtype of esophageal cancer in the US 50 years ago, esophageal adenocarcinoma (EAC) has surpassed it in prevalence in the US and western Europe, accounting for most new cases. The US incidence of EAC has increased at least sixfold since the 1970s and is projected to continue rising.[3] Barrett esophagus (BE), defined as intestinal metaplasia (IM) of the distal esophageal mucosa, typically results from chronic gastroesophageal reflux disease (GERD) and is the only known precursor of EAC. Patients with BE have a 30-fold to 125-fold increased risk of developing EAC compared with the general population[4]; the annual risk of BE progressing to EAC has been estimated between 0.1% and 0.5%.[5,6] Thus, BE is the link between GERD, the most common malady affecting the foregut, and EAC, the most rapidly increasing cancer in the western hemisphere.

The development of EAC is due to the malignant progression of BE through the intermediate steps of low-grade dysplasia (LGD) and high-grade dysplasia (HGD). Prevention of EAC can result by halting this progression at any point, by inducing regression, or by eradicating metaplastic or dysplastic esophageal mucosa. Screening and surveillance programs for BE have facilitated detection and treatment of metaplasia or dysplasia before the development of invasive malignancy, and before the onset of symptoms, allowing prophylactic or curative intervention. Unfortunately, only a small percentage of cases of EAC are detected by surveillance, highlighting the need both for an improved risk assessment tool for BE and for a cost-effective, patient-friendly screening tool that can be applied more widely than standard flexible endoscopy with biopsies.

As the development and progression of BE are related to GERD, medical and surgical antireflux therapies have been recommended to prevent EAC. In addition, endoscopic ablative and resective therapies have been popularized in recent years for the eradication of dysplastic BE or intramucosal EAC, largely replacing esophagectomy as the treatments of choice for these conditions. This article discusses the rationale behind these strategies and assesses their efficacy at preventing or curing EAC before the development of locoregionally advanced or systemic disease. Although chemopreventive therapies other than acid suppression have been investigated to reduce the esophageal cancer incidence in at-risk individuals, none yet have proven effective.

ANTIREFLUX THERAPIES FOR PREVENTION OF ESOPHAGEAL ADENOCARCINOMA
Medical Therapies

The development of BE results from injury to the normal distal esophageal squamous epithelium, usually due to the reflux of gastric juice including acid, bile salts, and enzymes, leading to mucosal regeneration with IM. Studies have estimated that 5% to 15% of individuals suffering from chronic GERD will develop BE.[7] Although White men are particularly susceptible, the reasons predisposing to the development of BE in a subset of refluxers, while sparing others, are poorly defined. The progression of IM to malignancy also is promoted by GERD. Given the role reflux plays in both the development and progression of BE, antireflux therapies are an obvious consideration in the prevention of EAC.

Contemporary medical therapy for GERD is targeted primarily at suppression of gastric acid production. Proton pump inhibitor (PPI) therapy, introduced in the in 1989, has been established as the most effective of the available medical regimens.

PPI therapy for chronic GERD, however, requires compliance with daily, or more frequent, dosing regimens often administered over years.

Several theories explain how PPIs could either prevent or promote the development of BE and EAC (**Table 1**). As chronic inflammation is a mechanism underlying tumorigenesis, and as PPIs can heal reflux esophagitis, PPI therapy might protect against the formation of esophageal cancer through anti-inflammatory effects on the esophageal lining. Acid has been shown to cause the production of reactive oxygen species, induce deoxyribonucleic acid damage, and promote cellular proliferation in BE, all of which can be carcinogenic; acid suppression counters these deleterious effects.[8,9] Finally, GERD has been shown to promote release of proinflammatory and cancer-promoting cytokines, such as interleukin-8, from the esophageal mucosa leading to cellular proliferation.[10] PPIs prevent cytokine release through a mechanism independent of acid suppression.[11]

Contrary to these protective effects, the potential role of PPIs in causing EAC is supported by several observations. Gastrin, secreted by gastric antral G cells in response to meals, stimulates acid production by gastric parietal cells. Acid, through a negative feedback loop, suppresses further gastrin production. As PPIs suppress gastric acid production, they interfere with this negative feedback loop and cause an increase in serum gastrin levels. Gastrin is known to promote cellular proliferation and reduce apoptosis in BE.

With the reduction of gastric acid caused by PPIs comes the potential for bacterial overgrowth in the stomach. Bacteria are known to deconjugate primary bile acids; the resultant deconjugates can injure the esophageal lining at neutral pH levels. Bacteria also promote the conversion of primary bile acids to noxious secondary bile acids, such as deoxycholic acid. Finally, bacteria can convert dietary nitrates into N-nitroso compounds. Both the secondary bile acids and these N-nitroso compounds are potentially carcinogenic to the esophageal mucosa.[12,13]

The impact of PPIs on the development of dysplasia or EAC in patients with BE has been investigated. Studies have found partial regression in the length of BE, particularly of short segments, with long-term PPI usage.[14,15] Partial regression, however, has not been associated with a decreased incidence of EAC. Other studies have shown PPIs to be associated with a reduction in the risk of BE progressing to dysplasia or EAC.[16–18]

Table 1
Mechanisms by which proton pump inhibitors might prevent or promote the development of esophageal adenocarcinoma

Potential Preventive Effects	Potential Causative Effects
Healing/prevention of reflux esophagitis	Increase in gastrin production by gastric antral G cells, leading to cellular proliferation and reduced apoptosis in the setting of BE
Reduction of reactive oxygen species, DNA damage, and cellular proliferation caused by GERD	
Prevention of the cytokine release from the esophageal mucosa that is induced by GERD	Promotion of gastric bacterial overgrowth, leading to development of proinflammatory or carcinogenic substrates via the following:
	• Deconjugation of primary bile acids
	• Conversion of primary bile acids to secondary bile acids
	• Conversion of dietary nitrates to N-nitroso compounds

Abbreviations: BE, Barrett esophagus; DNA, deoxyribonucleic acid; GERD, gastroesophageal reflux disease.

Contradictory results were obtained from a nationwide study in Denmark, however, which found patients adhering to PPI usage to have a higher chance of developing HGD and EAC than those who were nonadherent.[19] These results must be interpreted with caution, however, as patients requiring PPIs may have had more severe GERD; the refluxate, rather than PPIs, may have induced esophageal neoplasia.

A meta-analysis published in 2014 included 7 observational studies totaling 2813 patients with BE and 317 with EAC.[20] The use of PPIs was associated with a 71% reduction in the development of HGD or EAC, with therapy >2 to 3 years seemingly more protective than shorter-term administration. To date, however, no prospective, randomized, controlled clinical trials have shown that PPIs reduce the risk of dysplasia or EAC in patients with BE.

Antireflux Surgery

Patients with GERD and BE have more acid and bile reflux, a higher prevalence of an incompetent lower esophageal sphincter (LES), an increased likelihood of a hiatal hernia, and greater impairment in esophageal body function compared with patients with GERD and no BE.[21,22] These factors make control of GERD a challenge in the presence of BE, as they are markers of advanced disease.

Since the introduction of open transabdominal "gastroplication" by Rudolph Nissen in 1956, and with subsequent modifications (including the laparoscopic approach first reported by Dallemagne in 1991), fundoplication has been the mainstay of surgical antireflux therapy for more than 60 years.[23] The operation restores competency of the intrinsic LES, including both its pressure and its length, particularly the length exposed to the positive pressure environment of the abdomen. Fundoplication also restores the normal anatomic relationships and geometry of the hiatus and esophagogastric junction (EGJ), including repair of a hiatal hernia, when present, and narrowing of the widened hiatus, juxtaposing the hiatal fibers to the LES. The angle of His also is maintained or restored, preserving the "flap valve" at the EGJ.

Unlike medical therapy, which acts through acid suppression alone, fundoplication forms a mechanical barrier against reflux of acid, bile, pancreatic enzymes, and other components of gastric juice that are potentially noxious, mutagenic, or carcinogenic to the esophageal mucosa. Accordingly, this barrier could be advantageous in preventing the development of BE and EAC compared with medical therapy. Surgery also eliminates the need for acid suppressive medications, thereby avoiding their potential carcinogenic effects on the esophageal mucosa, and may reduce the lifetime cost of GERD treatment, particularly for younger patients.[24] The possible symptomatic and cancer-preventive benefits of fundoplication must be weighed against the downsides of surgery, including perioperative costs, risks, and potential long-term side effects.

The outcomes of antireflux surgery have been assessed across several domains, the most common being relief from typical reflux symptoms. With respect to BE, the pertinent outcome measures following fundoplication are the frequency and extent of regression and, more importantly, prevention of progression along the IM/dysplasia/EAC continuum. As 20% to 25% of patients with BE have been found on postoperative esophageal pH monitoring to have excessive esophageal acid exposure, GERD can continue to promote mucosal progression toward EAC even after surgery.[25,26]

Several studies have analyzed the fate of both non-dysplastic and dysplastic BE following fundoplication.[25,27,28] The data, viewed in aggregate, show that histologic regression of IM and LGD occurs in a minority of patients, with short-segment BE (SSBE; ≤3 cm) more prone to regression than long-segment BE (LSBE; >3 cm). Progression of BE occurs in a small minority of patients, typically those with LSBE or in the setting of abnormal postoperative esophageal pH monitoring.

Additional studies, including small, randomized controlled trials and 2 large litera-ture reviews, have assessed whether antireflux surgery is superior to medical therapy in the prevention of EAC for patients with BE. A meta-analysis of patients treated for BE included 34 publications with a cumulative 4678 patient-years of follow-up in the group undergoing antireflux surgery, and 4906 patient-years of follow-up in those medically treated.[29] The incidence of EAC was similar in both groups (3.8 vs 5.3 can-cers per 1000 patient-years; P = .29, respectively). The difference in outcomes was even smaller when only studies within the prior 5 years, for which PPIs were the stan-dard medical therapy, were considered.

A systematic review published in 2007 included 25 articles analyzing a total of 996 patients with BE undergoing antireflux surgery and 700 receiving suppression.[30] The incidence of EAC was significantly lower in the surgical cohort (2.8 vs 6.3 cases per 1000 patient-years; P = .034). The investigators reported the difference was largely present in uncontrolled case series, suggesting a possible publication bias. When only controlled studies were considered, the differences between surgically and medi-cally treated patients were no longer significantly different (4.8 vs 6.5 cases per 1000 patient-years; P = .32). The probability of disease regression was significantly higher in the surgical cohort in both uncontrolled and controlled studies.

The investigators of both retrospective reviews concluded that the incidence of EAC in patients with BE was low, and that fundoplication was not superior to acid suppres-sion for prevention of EAC. Antireflux surgery should not be offered, therefore, solely as a cancer-preventive measure. As patients with BE often have symptoms that are difficult to control, antireflux surgery is an excellent option to bring about relief, partic-ularly in patients who are noncompliant with medications, require multiple daily doses, or wish to discontinue medical therapy due to its cost, inconvenience, or concerns about side effects.

ENDOLUMINAL THERAPIES FOR DYSPLASTIC BARRETT ESOPHAGUS AND SUPERFICIAL ESOPHAGEAL CANCER
Histology of the Esophageal Wall

To understand the rationale for endoscopic treatment of dysplastic BE and superficial EAC, the clinician must possess an in-depth understanding of the histology of the esophageal wall and the terminology for associated histopathologies. The deep border of the esophageal epithelium is its basement membrane (**Fig. 1**). Dysplasia (LGD/HGD) is neoplasia limited to the epithelium, not penetrating beyond its basement

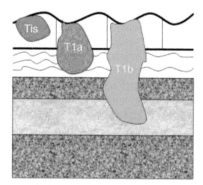

Epithelium

Lamina Propria

Muscularis mucosa

Submucosa

Muscularis propria

Fig. 1. Layers of the esophageal wall. Tis = in situ cancer = high-grade dysplasia; T1a = intramucosal carcinoma; T1b = submucosal carcinoma.

membrane. The term "carcinoma in situ" (CIS) is synonymous with HGD and Tis (American Joint Committee on Cancer, 8th edition staging).[31] Tumors invading beyond the basement membrane to involve the lamina propria or muscularis mucosa (MM) are classified as intramucosal carcinoma (IMC) or T1a lesions. Tumors invading beyond the MM are termed submucosal carcinoma (SMC) or T1b lesions. The submucosa has been further subdivided into even thirds (SM1/SM2/SM3) based on thickness as assessed on esophagectomy specimens.

Tumor penetration is important because the incidence of lymph node metastases, as assessed in esophagectomy specimens where a complete lymphadenectomy had been performed, correlates directly with increasing depth. Based on these data, 3 discrete subclassifications of superficial esophageal neoplasia have been defined:

1. Intraepithelial neoplasia (LGD, HGD/CIS/Tis) for which the risk of nodal spread is negligible
2. Intramucosal neoplasia (IMC, T1a) for which the risk of nodal spread is approximately 5%
3. Submucosal neoplasia (SMC, T1b) for which the risk of nodal spread is approximately 15% to 30%

Other factors besides tumor depth, such as tumor size, differentiation, and the presence of lymphovascular invasion (LVI), also are relevant in determining the potential for nodal disease. Based on these factors, a nomogram was created to stratify patients into low-risk ($\leq$2%), moderate-risk (3%–6%), and high-risk ($\geq$7%) groups for lymph node involvement.[32]

Endoluminal therapies are appropriate for esophageal neoplasia only when the absence of nodal metastases can be ensured with near certainty. For patients otherwise candidates for an esophagectomy, endoscopic eradication is indicated, therefore, in cases of dysplastic BE or IMC (T1a) where the risk of nodal spread is approximately 5% or less. Given the significantly higher risk of nodal disease in patients with SMC (T1b), most such cases should be treated with an esophagectomy and regional lymphadenectomy. Whether a select subgroup of submucosal tumors, such as those only superficially invading the submucosa (SM1), carry a low risk of nodal spread and are eligible for endoscopic treatment has been investigated.[33] Additional study on larger cohorts of patients is necessary before an endoscopic treatment paradigm can be considered standard of care for such tumors. In patients deemed high risk for esophagectomy, endoscopic resection (ER) may be reasonable for SMC, accepting the risk of untreated nodal disease and its potential for dissemination.

Considerable interobserver variability exists in the histopathologic interpretation of ER specimens in the setting of BE and early neoplasia, particularly relative to the depth of tumor penetration.[34,35] Given the major impact such determinations have on predicting the risk of lymph node metastases and subsequent therapeutic recommendations, the need for reliable review and consensus cannot be overemphasized. Analysis of biopsies by an expert gastrointestinal pathologist should be undertaken routinely, even if the specimens must be sent outside of the home institution for assessment.

Pretreatment Evaluation

A comprehensive endoscopic evaluation of the entire esophageal mucosa is mandatory in patients with BE before endoscopic ablation or resection. Esophageal mucosal abnormalities may be subtle, requiring a thorough examination by an experienced endoscopist. Adjuncts to standard white light endoscopy, including high-resolution endoscopy, narrow band imaging, chromoendoscopy with vital stains, or confocal laser endomicroscopy, should be considered to enhance detection of mucosal pathology.[36]

Current standards of care mandate 4-quadrant biopsies every 2 cm along the length of suspected BE, as per the "Seattle protocol," for a minimum of 8 biopsies.[37] In cases of documented dysplasia, 4-quadrant biopsies should be obtained every 1 cm. In addition, focused biopsies should be performed of any regions containing mucosal nodularity or irregularity. In this fashion, the esophageal mucosa is "mapped" before initiating treatment.

Endoscopic ultrasound (EUS) has been instrumental in evaluating esophageal tumors relative to their depth of invasion and the presence of regional lymphadenopathy. Tumor depth and nodal involvement are erroneously interpreted on EUS in 45% and 25% of cases, respectively.[38] The reliability of EUS is highest in differentiating T1 and T2 tumors from deeper T3 or T4 disease. The accuracy of EUS in differentiating Tis versus T1a versus T1b tumors is low, despite the introduction of high-frequency (20 MHz) mini-probes designed to improve the assessment of superficial tumor depth. The accuracy of high-frequency EUS for determining mucosal involvement is approximately 90%, but is only approximately 50% for detecting submucosal invasion.[36,39] Considering the limited accuracy of EUS in identifying submucosal disease, ER is mandatory to allow histologic evaluation of tumor depth in all cases of small, discrete, esophageal nodules. The depth of invasion of superficial tumors is assessed best under a microscope, in which determinations measured in microns, and involving landmarks smaller than the resolution of EUS, can be made.

Endoscopic Resection

The term "ER" is synonymous with the term "EMR" (endoscopic mucosal resection), the latter being a misnomer in that both submucosa and mucosa typically are removed in the specimen. Endoscopic submucosal dissection has arisen as an alternative to ER, although is a more technically demanding procedure for which fewer outcomes data are available. This discussion will focus on data specific to ER.

The use of ER as definitive therapy for early esophageal cancer was first introduced in Japan. Initially intended for cure of superficial esophageal squamous cell carcinoma, ER was adopted in western countries for treatment of BE with HGD or IMC. The use of ER accomplishes 2 valuable goals in the setting of nodular BE. First, it provides a generous specimen, superior to standard endoscopic biopsies, for evaluation of tumor depth, differentiation, grade, the presence of LVI, and the status of the lateral and deep resection margins, which can guide subsequent definitive therapy. Second, used alone or in combination with endoscopic ablation of surrounding metaplasia and dysplasia, ER offers curative treatment of small tumors that carry a low risk of nodal or distant metastatic spread, such as those confined to the epithelium or mucosa. Although ER has been used to remove large areas of BE, circumferential resections should be avoided as they cause stricturing.[40]

Over the past 15 years, ER has become a standard of care for eradication of IMC, largely supplanting esophagectomy. In 2007, Ell and colleagues[41] reported a 99% local remission rate, a 98% 5-year survival, no severe complications, and no cancer deaths in 100 patients with "low-risk" IMC treated with ER (**Box 1**). A follow-up study assessed a cohort of 1000 patients with T1a EAC.[42] Long-term complete remission and overall 5-year survival were observed in 93.8% and 91.5%, respectively, confirming the efficacy of ER in this setting.

Given its favorable complication profile, quick postprocedural recovery, and short hospital stay, ER is associated with numerous advantages over esophagectomy. The data assessing ER in appropriately selected cases of early esophageal neoplasia

---

Box 1
Indications for endoscopic resection in the setting of esophageal adenocarcinoma

- Lesion ≤20 mm
- Polypoid or flat
- Well to moderately differentiated
- Tumor limited to mucosa
- Negative deep resection margin
- No lymphovascular invasion
- No lymph node involvement or systemic metastases on staging

Modified from: Ell C, May A, Pech O, et al. Curative endoscopic resection of early esophageal adenocarcinoma (Barrett's cancer). Gastrointest Endosc 2007;65:3-10.

---

show cure rates equivalent to esophageal resection but with less morbidity. The excellent outcomes reported in these case series are the result of rigorous and accurate pretreatment evaluation, skilled endoscopic intervention, expert pathologic assessment, and careful patient follow-up using established protocols. In choosing a course of endoscopic therapy, both the patient and their treating physician must be committed to the serial endoscopies required for ongoing evaluation, therapy, and subsequent surveillance, typically occurring over the course of years.

Endoscopic Ablation

Several endoscopic ablative technologies have arisen for eradication of BE, the most commonly used being radiofrequency ablation (RFA); others include cryotherapy, photodynamic therapy (PDT), argon plasma coagulation (APC), and multipolar electro-coagulation. Although each modality has its pros and cons, all ablative technologies share the goal of necrosing pathologic esophageal mucosa so that it can be replaced by normal squamous epithelium. Protection against acid reflux, using either acid suppression medications or antireflux surgery, is an essential adjunct to prevent recurrence of IM.

Both circumferential and focal RFA devices are available (Medtronic, Minneapolis, MN). They deliver high power (300 W) at a preset energy density over a short time (<300 ms), leading to a thermal burn with a controlled depth of penetration (approximately 500 μm to 700 μm) limited to the MM. As injury to the submucosa generally is avoided, postprocedural esophageal stricturing is uncommon. The indications for RFA are listed in **Box 2**. After a thorough endoscopic inspection, consideration should

---

Box 2
Indications for radiofrequency ablation in Barrett esophagus

- High-grade dysplasia
- Low-grade dysplasia, confirmed on at least 2 biopsies 6 weeks apart and with adequate acid suppression therapy in the interim
- Nondysplastic intestinal metaplasia after endoscopic resection of intramucosal cancer or focal dysplasia

---

be given to ER of any nodular lesions to rule out EAC invading into the submucosa. Also, because of its limited depth of tissue injury, RFA is most effective on smooth BE. A delay of 6 to 8 weeks typically is recommended after ER before performing RFA.

The technique of RFA has been described in numerous publications. After ablation, the patient is kept on a twice-daily PPI regimen to prevent regrowth of IM. Esophageal stricturing is the most frequent complication following RFA, although occurs in only approximately 6% of cases and is generally mild and easily treated.[43,44] Hemorrhage and perforation are rare, occurring in less than 1% of cases. Adverse events associated with RFA are fourfold higher when ER previously was performed.

Follow-up ablations are scheduled every 2 to 3 months until complete eradication (CE) of IM has been obtained. The optimal surveillance interval following CE has not been established, although serial endoscopies every 3 months for the first year, every 6 months for the second year, and yearly thereafter seem reasonable if IM does not recur. The minimum duration of surveillance has not been determined.

An extensive literature has assessed the outcomes following RFA for nondysplastic and dysplastic BE. From a randomized, sham-controlled, prospective clinical trial of RFA for dysplastic BE, an intention-to-treat analysis at 12 months of follow-up found CE of IM in 77%, CE of LGD in 91%, and CE of HGD in 81% of those undergoing ablation.[43] Disease progression occurred in 3.6% of treated patients, and progression to cancer occurred in 1.2%. In a follow-up of this same patient cohort, the rate of EAC development was 1 per 181 patient-years (0.55%/patient-year), although no cases of cancer-related morbidity or mortality were detected.[45]

A systematic review and meta-analysis of RFA for BE revealed CE of IM in 78%, CE of dysplasia in 91%, and progression to EAC in 0.2% of patients following treatment.[46] When CE of IM was achieved, EAC subsequently arose in 0.7%. A retrospective cohort study assessed 306 patients who had undergone RFA for dysplastic BE and had achieved a CE for IM.[47] Over more than 540.6 person-years of follow-up, 1.8% of cases progressed to EAC. Longer segments of BE were at higher risk for developing cancer than shorter segments. In a review of the US multicenter RFA Patient Registry, 100 (2%) of 4892 patients developed EAC with 9 EAC-related deaths.[48] Multivariate logistic regression analysis found baseline BE length and baseline histology (odds ratios, 5.8 and 50.3 for LGD and HGD, respectively) predictive of progression to EAC.

Although RFA is a highly effective therapy for BE with or without dysplasia, several factors have correlated with an unsuccessful outcome. Incomplete eradication of BE at 3 months following initial ablation has been associated with overall treatment failure or the need for a prolonged treatment course.[49] Incomplete mucosal healing between treatment sessions, LSBE, uncontrolled acid reflux, a large hiatal hernia, advanced age, and non-Caucasian race have been identified as additional predictors of incomplete eradication of IM or increased recurrence risk.[50] The most likely location of recurrent IM is the esophagogastric junction.[51] This finding suggests that biopsies directed just beyond the squamocolumnar junction are imperative at the time of endoscopic surveillance. The potential for IM "buried" beneath neo-squamous epithelium must be considered as well, as it can lead to treatment failure.[52] Cases have been reported of EAC developing in "subsquamous" IM after ablation.[53]

Endoscopic Ablation Following Endoscopic Resection

Although ER is targeted at discrete esophageal mucosal nodules, cases of HGD or EAC usually occur in the setting of surrounding IM. As this metaplastic mucosa is at-risk for malignant progression, the concept of eradicating it holds appeal. Based on the extensive experience from Ell and colleagues[41] in Germany with ER for mucosal EAC, rates of recurrent or metachronous neoplasia were increased when use of adjunctive endoscopic ablation was decreased. In their report from 2007,[41] endoscopic ablation (typically with APC for SSBE or PDT for LSBE) was used in 49 (49%) of 100 cases and the rate of recurrent or metachronous neoplasia was 11% at a mean follow-up of 36.7 months. In a subsequent publication from 2008 analyzing 349 patients, their use of endoscopic ablation had decreased to 20% of cases. The incidence of recurrent or metachronous cancer increased to 21.5%, although at a longer mean follow-up of 63.6 months.[54] Additional studies are needed to understand the utility of endoscopic ablation as an adjunct to ER for early esophageal neoplasia.

SUMMARY

The incidence of EAC continues to rise in the United States and western Europe, a trend that has been observed for more than 40 years. Despite improvements in cancer care, EAC carries a poor prognosis, largely due its advanced stage at the typical time of diagnosis. Until better systemic therapies are developed, EAC must be prevented or treated early in its course to improve survival. As BE is a known precursor to EAC, and as both the development and progression of BE are related to GERD, antireflux therapies play a role not only in symptom relief but also in cancer prevention. Although antireflux surgery has not proven superior to acid suppression therapy in preventing EAC, it is an excellent option for control of symptoms in patients with BE, who frequently suffer the manifestations of severe reflux disease. Antireflux surgery also obviates the need for patient compliance with medical therapy, which commonly requires lifelong treatment in daily or more frequent doses. In cases in which dysplastic BE or superficial EAC has arisen, endoscopic therapies have been developed for eradication of esophageal mucosal disease before progression to locoregionally advanced malignancy. Appropriate utilization of these endoscopic techniques may lead to avoidance of esophagectomy in many cases for which it previously was indicated.

The standard of care for the management of early esophageal neoplasia in the setting of BE has changed drastically over the past 15 years. Further investigation into diagnostic and therapeutic adjuncts will continue to improve our ability to control or cure BE before its advancement to a life-threatening malignancy.

CLINICS CARE POINTS

- Barrett esophagus (BE) is intestinal metaplasia of the distal esophageal mucosa and results from chronic gastroesophageal reflux disease (GERD).
- Esophageal adenocarcinoma (EAC) arises from the progression of BE through the intermediate steps of low-grade and high-grade dysplasia
- As GERD is implicated both in the development of BE and its progression to EAC, control of GERD with acid suppressive medications or antireflux surgery can help prevent EAC.
- Endoscopic resection and ablation can treat dysplastic BE and superficial EAC prior to the development of advanced malignancy and have largely replaced esophagectomy for these indications.
- EAC continues to increase in incidence and carries a poor prognosis, largely attributable to its common presentation in an advanced stage and the lack of effective systemic therapies against it.
- Survival from EAC, therefore, is dependent on early detection and treatment.

REFERENCES

1. American Cancer Society. Cancer facts and figures 2020. Atlanta, GA: American Cancer Society; 2020. accessed August 6, 2020.
2. National Cancer Institute. Surveillance, epidemiology, and end results program. 2020. Available at: seer.cancer.gov. Accessed August 23, 2020.
3. Simard EP, Ward EM, Siegel R, et al. Cancers with increasing incidence trends in the United States: 1999 through 2008. CA Cancer J Clin 2012;62:118–28.
4. Cameron AJ, Ott BJ, Payne WS. The incidence of adenocarcinoma in columnar-lined (Barrett's) esophagus. N Engl J Med 1985;313(14):857–9.
5. Hvid-Jensen F, Pedersen L, Drewes AM, et al. Incidence of adenocarcinoma among patients with Barrett's esophagus. N Engl J Med 2011;365(15):1375–83.
6. Bhat S, Coleman HG, Yousef F, et al. Risk of malignant progression in Barrett's esophagus patient: results from a large population-based study. J Natl Cancer Inst 2011;103(13):1049–57.
7. Shaheen NJ, Richter JE. Barrett's oesophagus. Lancet 2009;373(9666):850–61.
8. Zhang HY, Hormi-Carver K, Zhang X, et al. In benign Barrett's epithelial cells, acid exposure generates reactive oxygen species that cause DNA double-strand breaks. Cancer Res 2009;69(23):9083–9.
9. Fitzgerald RC, Omary MB, Triadafilopoulos G. Dynamic effects of acid on Barrett's esophagus. An ex vivo proliferation and differentiation model. J Clin Invest 1996;98(9):2120–8.
10. Souza RF, Huo X, Mittal V, et al. Gastroesophageal reflux might cause esophagitis through a cytokine-mediated mechanism rather than caustic acid injury. Gastroenterology 2009;137(5):1776–84.
11. Huo X, Zhang X, Yu C, et al. In oesophageal squamous cells exposed to acidic bile salt medium, omeprazole inhibits IL-8 expression through effects on nuclear factor-kappa B and activator protein-1. Gut 2014;63(7):1042–52.
12. Peng S, Huo X, Rezaei D, et al. In Barrett's esophagus patients and Barrett's cell lines, ursodeoxycholic acid increases antioxidant expression and prevents DNA damage by bile acids. Am J Physiol Gastrointest Liver Physiol 2014;307(2):G129–39.
13. Williams C, McColl KE. Review article: proton pump inhibitors and bacterial overgrowth. Aliment Pharmacol Ther 2006;23(1):3–10.
14. Srinivasan R, Katz PO, Ramakrishnan A, et al. Maximal acid reflux control for Barrett's oesophagus: feasible and effective. Aliment Pharmacol Ther 2001;15(4):519–24.
15. Cooper BT, Chapman W, Neumann CS, et al. Continuous treatment of Barrett's oesophagus patients with proton pump inhibitors up to 13 years: observations on regression and cancer incidence. Aliment Pharmacol Ther 2006;23(6):727–33.
16. El-Serag HB, Aguirre TV, Davis S, et al. Proton pump inhibitors are associated with reduced incidence of dysplasia in Barrett's esophagus. Am J Gastroenterol 2004;99(10):1877–83.
17. Nguyen DM, El-Serag HB, Henderson L, et al. Medication usage and the risk of neoplasia in patients with Barrett's esophagus. Clin Gastroenterol Hepatol 2009;7(12):199–304.
18. Kastelein F, Spaander MC, Steyerberg EW, et al. Proton pump inhibitors reduce the risk of neoplastic progression in patients with Barrett's esophagus. Clin Gastroenterol Hepatol 2013;11(4):382–8.
19. Hvid-Jensen F, Pedersen L, Funch-Jensen P, et al. Proton pump inhibitor use may not prevent high-grade dysplasia and oesophageal adenocarcinoma in Barrett's

oesophagus: a nationwide study of 9883 patients. Aliment Pharmacol Ther 2014; 39(9):984–91.

20. Singh S, Garg SK, Singh PP, et al. Acid-suppressive medications and risk of oesophageal adenocarcinoma in patients with Barrett's oesophagus: a systematic review and meta-analysis. Gut 2014;63(8):1229–37.

21. Cameron AJ. Barrett's esophagus: prevalence and size of hiatal hernia. Am J Gastroenterol 1999;94(8):2054–9.

22. Avidan B, Sonnenberg A, Schnell TG, et al. Hiatal hernia size, Barrett's length, and severity of acid reflux are all risk factors for esophageal adenocarcinoma. Am J Gastroenterol 2002;97(8):1930–6.

23. Stylopoulos N, Rattner DW. The history of hiatal hernia surgery: from Bowditch to laparoscopy. Ann Surg 2005;241(1):185–93.

24. Gawron AJ, French DD, Pandolfino JE, et al. Economic evaluations of gastroesophageal reflux disease medical management: a systematic review. Pharmacoeconomics 2014;32(8):745–58.

25. Oelschlager BK, Barreca M, Chang L, et al. Clinical and pathologic response of Barrett's esophagus to laparoscopic antireflux surgery. Ann Surg 2003;238(4): 458–64 [discussion: 464–6].

26. Hofstetter WL, Peters JH, DeMeester TR, et al. Long-term outcome of antireflux surgery in patients with Barrett's esophagus. Ann Surg 2001;234(4):532–8 [discussion: 538–9].

27. O'Riordan JM, Byrne PJ, Ravi N, et al. Long-term clinical and pathologic response of Barrett's esophagus after antireflux surgery. Am J Surg 2004; 188(1):27–33.

28. Gurski RR, Peters JH, Hagen JA, et al. Barrett's esophagus can and does regress after antireflux surgery: a study of prevalence and predictive features. J Am Coll Surg 2003;196(5):706–12 [discussion: 712–3].

29. Corey KE, Schmitz SM, Shaheen NJ. Does a surgical antireflux procedure decrease the incidence of esophageal adenocarcinoma in Barrett's esophagus? A meta-analysis. Am J Gastroenterol 2003;98(11):2390–4.

30. Chang EY, Morris CD, Seltman AK, et al. The effect of antireflux surgery on esophageal carcinogenesis in patients with Barrett esophagus: a systematic review. Ann Surg 2007;246(1):11–21.

31. Amin MB, Edge S, Greene F, et al, editors. AJCC cancer staging manual. 8th edition. Springer International Publishing: American Joint Commission on Cancer; 2017.

32. Lee L, Ronellenfitsch U, Hofstetter WL, et al. Predicting lymph node metastases in early esophageal adenocarcinoma using a simple scoring system. J Am Coll Surg 2013;217(2):191–9.

33. Manner H, May A, Pech O, et al. Early Barrett's carcinoma with "low-risk" submucosal invasion: long-term results of endoscopic resection with a curative intent. Am J Gastroenterol 2008;103:2589–97.

34. Ormsby AH, Petras RE, Henricks WH, et al. Observer variation in the diagnosis of superficial esophageal adenocarcinoma. Gut 2002;51:671–6.

35. Montgomery E, Bronner MP, Goldblum JR, et al. Reproducibility of the diagnosis of dysplasia in Barrett esophagus: a reaffirmation. Hum Pathol 2001;32:368–78.

36. May A. Accuracy of staging in early oesophageal cancer using high resolution endoscopy and high resolution endosonography: a comparative, prospective, and blinded trial. Gut 2004;53(5):634–40.

37. Shaheen NJ, Falk GW, Iyer PG, et al. ACG clinical guideline: diagnosis and management of Barrett's esophagus. Am J Gastroenterol 2016;111:30–50.

38. Pech O, Günter E, Dusemund F, et al. Accuracy of endoscopic ultrasound in pre-operative staging of esophageal cancer: results from a referral center for early esophageal cancer. Endoscopy 2010;42(06):456–61.
39. Chemaly M, Scalone O, Durivage G, et al. Miniprobe EUS in the pretherapeutic assessment of early esophageal neoplasia. Endoscopy 2007;40(1):2–6.
40. van Vilsteren FGI, Pouw RE, Seewald S, et al. Stepwise radical endoscopic resection versus radiofrequency ablation for Barrett's oesophagus with high-grade dysplasia or early cancer: a multicentre randomised trial. Gut 2011;60(6):765–73.
41. Ell C, May A, Pech O, et al. Curative endoscopic resection of early esophageal adenocarcinoma (Barrett's cancer). Gastrointest Endosc 2007;65:3–10.
42. Pech O, May A, Manner H, et al. Long-term efficacy and safety of endoscopic resection for patients with mucosal adenocarcinoma of the esophagus. Gastroenterology 2014;146(3):652–60.
43. Shaheen NJ, Sharma P, Overholt BF, et al. Radiofrequency ablation in Barrett's esophagus with dysplasia. N Engl J Med 2009;360:2277–88.
44. Luigiano C, Iabichino G, Eusebi LH, et al. Outcomes of radiofrequency ablation for dysplastic Barrett's esophagus: a comprehensive review. Gastroenterol Res Pract 2016;2016:1–8.
45. Shaheen NJ, Overholt BF, Sampliner RE, et al. Durability of radiofrequency ablation in Barrett's esophagus with dysplasia. Gastroenterology 2011;141:460–8.
46. Orman ES, Li N, Shaheen NJ, et al. Efficacy and durability of radiofrequency ablation for Barrett's esophagus: a systematic review and meta-analysis. Clin Gastroenterol Hepatol 2013;11:1245–55.
47. Guthikonda A, Cotton CC, Madanick RD, et al. Clinical outcomes following recurrence of intestinal metaplasia after successful treatment of Barrett's esophagus with radiofrequency ablation. Am J Gastroenterol 2016;112(1):87–94.
48. Wolf WA, Pasricha S, Cotton C, et al. Incidence of esophageal adenocarcinoma and causes of mortality after radiofrequency ablation of Barrett's esophagus. Gastroenterology 2015;149(7):1752–62.
49. van Vilsteren F, Alvarez-Herrero L, Pouw R, et al. Predictive factors for initial treatment response after circumferential radiofrequency ablation for Barrett's esophagus with early neoplasia: a prospective multicenter study. Endoscopy 2013;45(7):516–25.
50. Krishnan K, Pandolfino JE, Kahrilas PJ, et al. Increased risk for persistent intestinal metaplasia in patients with Barrett's esophagus and uncontrolled reflux exposure before radiofrequency ablation. Gastroenterology 2012;143(3):576–81.
51. Cotton CC, Wolf WA, Pasricha S, et al. Recurrent intestinal metaplasia after radiofrequency ablation for Barrett's esophagus: endoscopic findings and anatomic location. Gastrointest Endosc 2015;81(6):1362–9.
52. Komatsu Y, Landreneau R, Jobe BA. Buried Barrett metaplasia after endoluminal ablation: a ticking time bomb or much ado about nothing? J Gastrointest Surg 2017;21(2):249–50.
53. Lee JK, Cameron RG, Binmoeller KF, et al. Recurrence of subsquamous dysplasia and carcinoma after successful endoscopic and radiofrequency ablation therapy for dysplastic Barrett's esophagus. Endoscopy 2013;45(7):571–4.
54. Pech O, Behrens A, May A, et al. Long-term results and risk factor analysis for recurrence after curative endoscopic therapy in 349 patients with high-grade intraepithelial neoplasia and mucosal adenocarcinoma in Barrett's oesophagus. Gut 2008;57:1200–6.

Staging of Esophageal Malignancy

Ealaf Shemmeri, MD[a],*, Thomas Fabian, MD[b]

KEYWORDS

- Esophageal cancer • Staging of esophageal cancer • Esophageal cancer work-up

KEY POINTS

- Esophageal staging leads to better treatment and improved patient outcomes.
- Avoiding over-staging or under-staging in esophageal cancer is critical.
- Esophageal staging is paramount to maximizing outcomes.

INTRODUCTION

Esophageal cancer will claim more than 16,000 deaths in the United States (2020), with a lifetime risk of 1 in 125 men and 1 in 417 women. Worldwide, a majority of these tumors are squamous cell carcinoma. In the United States, where the most common histology is adenocarcinoma, esophageal cancer accounts for 1% of all cancers. Historically, 5-year survival was dismal, at approximately 5%, but this has increased to 20% for all patients. The Surveillance, Epidemiology, and End Results database from 2009 to 2015 shows early-stage esophageal cancers have the highest 5-year survival, at 47%. Those with regional disease have 25% survival and those with metastatic disease have a 5-year survival of 5% (National Comprehensive Cancer Network [NCCN]).[1] The stark survival difference between those patients with early disease and regional disease makes it paramount to promptly diagnose and start stage-specific treatment of patients.

Staging of esophageal cancer is determined by the TNM classification system, with the most recent edition in use since 2018 (*AJCC Cancer Staging Manual*, 8th edition).[2–4] T represents tumor, N lymph nodes, and M metastasis and is independent of histologic cell type (**Table 1**).

Esophageal cancer also is described based on anatomic location; this has implications for optimal treatment options and prognosis. There are 5 anatomic areas. The cervical esophagus is from the oropharynx to the sternal notch (15–20 cm from the

[a] Section of Thoracic Surgery, Department of Surgery, Albany Medical College, 3rd Floor, 50 New Scotland Avenue, Albany, NY 12208, USA; [b] Section of Thoracic Surgery, Albany Medical College, 47 New Scotland Avenue, Albany, NY 12208, USA
* Corresponding author.
E-mail address: shemmee@amc.edu

Surg Clin N Am 101 (2021) 405–414
https://doi.org/10.1016/j.suc.2021.03.003
0039-6109/21/© 2021 Elsevier Inc. All rights reserved.

surgical.theclinics.com

Table 1
Clinical staging for esophageal cancer

	Squamous Cell Carcinoma			Adenocarcinoma
Stage 1	T1	N0/N1	M0	T1N1M0
Stage 2	T2	N0/N1	M0	2a = T1N1M0
				2b = T2N0M0
Stage 3	T1/T2	N2	M0	T2N1M0
	T3	N1/N2	M0	T3/T4a N0/N1 M0
Stage 4	T4a/T4b Any T Any T	N0/N1/N2	M0	4a = T1-T4a N2M0
		N3	M0	T4bN0/N 1/N2M0
		Any N	M1	Any TN3M0
				4b = Any T Any N M1

Used with permission of the American College of Surgeons, Chicago, Illinois. The original source for this information is the AJCC Cancer Staging System (2020).

incisors), the upper esophagus is from the sternal notch to the lower border of the azygous vein (20–25 cm), the middle esophagus is from the azygous vein to the lower border of the inferior pulmonary veins (25–30 cm), the lower esophagus is from the inferior pulmonary veins to the stomach (30–40 cm),[4] and finally the gastroesophageal junction.

The most common symptom of esophageal cancer is dysphagia. In addition to history and physical examination, dysphagia should be evaluated with endoscopy and/or esophagram. If concern of cancer is high, esophagoscopy is critical and can establish the diagnosis. Once malignancy is confirmed, the staging evaluation can begin. Half of patients with esophageal cancer present with advanced or metastatic disease.[1] Formal staging is required and is directed at confirmation of the tumor thickness, nodal involvement, and presence of metastasis that make up the TNM staging classification.

CLINICAL STAGING
T Staging

Tumor invasion occurs longitudinally as well as radially within the esophageal wall. Early lesions range from in situ with dysplasia to invasion into the submucosal layer. The current nomenclature is Tis (carcinoma in situ), T1a to describe mucosal invasion, and T1b for submucosal invasion. When discussing these layers in more depth, subcategories describe the layers even further. The exact depth of invasion for either squamous cell carcinoma or adenocarcinoma dictates substantial differences in survival. Historic esophagectomy data for early esophageal cancer reflect the aggressive nature of this tumor. Ancona and colleagues[5] reviewed 98 esophagectomy patients with superficial cancer (Tis, T1a, and T1b). They stratified the histology into mucosal: m1, m2, or m3, or submucosa: sm1, sm2, or sm3, for further histologic assessment of invasion. With a median of 15 lymph nodes sampled on the esophagectomy specimens, they found that tumors limited to the mucosa had no lymph nodes involved, whereas 28% of submucosal tumors (T1b) had metastasis to lymph nodes. Metastasis was rare in T1b tumors, but 4 patients' final pathology demonstrated distant metastasis in the liver, lung, pulmonary vein, and celiac trunk. Multivariate analysis showed that lymphocytic infiltration and neural invasion along with the depth involvement significantly added to the development of lymph node metastasis. Five-year survival rates were 77.7% for T1m (T1a) and 53.3% for T1sm (T1b) ($P = .048$). With such a stark difference in survival, accurate T staging alters the choice of treatment strategies (**Table 2**).

To evaluate the depth of early cancer, the authors rely on esophagoscopy and advanced endoscopic instruments, including endomucosal resection (EMR) and endoscopic ultrasound (EUS). Diagnostic testing of T stage commences with esophagoscopy. This evaluation tool establishes a general road map of how the native esophagus looks (longitudinal length of tumor and presence of Barrett's disease), morphology of the cancer (fungating and obstructing), and what anatomic portion is affected (distance from the incisors).

Advanced endoscopic techniques include EMR, which resects a specific area in the esophagus, including the mucosal layer. An endoscope is placed in proximity to the tumor and the lesion either is elevated using hydrodissection or suctioned into the end cap of the endoscope and then snared and removed. This method can provide more substantial tissue quantity than traditional biopsy specimens. It is effective in differentiating T status of early tumors, and it can act as a therapeutic resection of early cancerous lesions confined to the mucosal layer. If histopathologic margins are negative, no further treatment is needed. This technique has revolutionized the management of high-grade dysplasia and of T1 lesions and is discussed at length in an earlier article. EMR is very accurate for staging of esophageal cancer. Hofstetter[6] evaluated EMR accuracy and described the technique as the most accurate modality available for T1 cancers, better than EUS.

EUS generally is considered standard in the work-up for esophageal cancer. EUS has gone through multiple advancements with regard to the size of the circular probe, the frequency of its depth analysis, and the ability to be used within a narrowed lumen. Early data in staging esophageal cancer yielded varying accuracy in the literature. Differences in the specificity and sensitivity are thought to be due to the location of the tumors, histologic type, high-frequency hertz versus traditional hertz, and interoperator variability.[7–12]

A meta-analysis by Thosani and colleagues[8] reviewed 19 studies on EUS in staging. EUS, compared with EMR and surgical resection, was analyzed to find the sensitivity and specificity in pathologic staging. For T1a tumors, EUS had a sensitivity ratio of 0.85 (95% CI, 0.82–0.88) and specificity of 0.87 (95%, CI, 0.84–0.90). For T1b lesions, the sensitivity ratio was 0.86 (95% CI, 0.82–0.89) and specificity was 0.86 (95% CI, 0.83–0.89). The investigators found an overall accuracy, as area under the curve, of greater than 0.93 for combined T1a and T1b lesions. They included data from variable studies using standard and high-frequency EUS probes, EUS miniprobes, squamous and adenocarcinoma histology, and tumors of distal and nondistal esophagus. As a staging tool for early cancers, EUS fares well. As the higher-frequency probes become more widespread in use and the literature, EUS accuracy may improve.

For early cancers (Tis, T1a, and T1b), PET/computed tomography (CT) scan is not useful. Cuellar and colleagues[13] reviewed 79 patients with early adenocarcinoma staged with endoscopy and EUS, all of whom had preoperative PET/CT scans. Four

Table 2			
Early esophageal cancer and rates of N and M for each depth			
T Stage	Depth of Invasion	N (%)	M (%)
Tis (m1)	Mucosa	0	0
T1a (m2 and m3)	Mucosal to submucosa	5	0.04
T1b (sm1-sm2-sm3)	Submucosa	28	

patients had false-positive M1 lesions. None of the subgroup analyses showed PET scan avidity correlating with predicting pathologic T stage in this cohort. Additionally, 1 in 5 patients had a delay in treatment as a result of undergoing PET scan testing; therefore, the investigators concluded there is no utility to evaluating early cancers with PET/CT scan.

T2 lesions are defined as those that have traversed the submucosa into the muscularis propria. Once tumors invade into the lymphovascular plexus between the submucosal and inner circular muscularis layer, the spread of tumor cells is easy and bidirectional.[14] T3 tumors invade the adventitia surrounding the muscular wall of the esophagus and T4 tumors invade neighboring structures, such as pleura, pericardium, azygos vein, diaphragm, and peritoneum. T4b tumor subclassification is reserved for invasion into the aorta, vertebral body, or trachea.[4]

Locally advanced disease can include airway invasion. This becomes more relevant in more proximal esophageal cancers. For tumors involving the proximal and middle thirds of the esophagus, staging should include bronchoscopy. Bronchoscopy with visualization and biopsies, if necessary, are critical to rule out invasion of the airway (T4 disease).

For advanced obstructing lesions that are too tight to traverse with endoscopy, either double-contrast barium esophagram or CT scan with oral and intravenous (IV) contrast (chest/abdomen/pelvis) can be used selectively as the initial test to allow for staging. With newer testing available, esophagram and CT scan are needed less frequently and, when ordering these tests, concerns regarding aspiration must be addressed. Generally, the esophagram is performed with the patient upright. For healthy patients, this is safe if they can step onto the table or step off the table. For more infirm patients, they often are placed supine at the conclusion of the procedure, exposing them to risk. Previously in this article, clinical assessment is discussed. Generally speaking, patients who present with significant dysphagia are T2 or higher, and bulky tumors seen on CT scan indicate T3 tumors. In certain circumstances, that clinical intuition to identify advanced lesions may be adequate to start treatment planning.

N Staging

N staging includes regional nodes extending from the supraclavicular region down to paragastric/celiac nodes and is based on the number of affected nodes present. N1 is the presence of fewer than 3 nodes involved with cancer. N2 is the presence of 3 to 6 nodes, and N3 is more than 7 nodes harboring cancer (**Box 1**).

The most challenging staging is the N status in esophageal cancer. Although physical examination may reveal palpable cervical or umbilical nodes, it does not inform of paraesophageal nodal status of the patient. There are no specific tools geared toward lymph node identification. The authors currently have established EUS, CT scan, and PET/CT scan for N staging. Arguably, the best of these modalities for N staging is EUS. Only EUS can identify enlarged nodes and sample them with fine-needle aspiration (FNA) to confirm or refute malignancy. False-positive results and false-negative results

Box 1	
Esophageal cancer lymph node staging	
N1	<3 lymph nodes involved
N2	3–6 nodes involved
N3	≥7 lymph nodes involved

exist in both PET and CT, and other studies, frequently EUS, are relied on to determine pathologic status of suspicious lymph nodes. Yet, there lies significant controversy in the literature regarding the accuracy of EUS in lymph node staging, even with the addition of FNA. This becomes problematic because the clinical staging greatly affects the treatment and, ultimately, the overall survival of patients with esophageal cancer. Lymph node metastasis shortens overall survival dramatically and is associated with early development of distant disease.

Several institutions have presented their discordant clinical and pathologic T2N0 data. The Memorial Sloan Kettering group recently reviewed outcomes in clinical T2N0 patients.[7] A total of 72 patients staged as cT2N0 with the use of PET/CT scan and EUS underwent esophagectomy. Pathologic evaluation of lymph nodes segregated the cohort into those with and those without lymph node metastasis of their cancer. Despite 28 (35%) patients having lymph node metastasis on their final pathology, their index tumor PET standardized uptake value (SUV) was similar to those who had no lymph node involvement (SUV 6.2 vs SUV 4; $P = .24$). EUS was inaccurate in predicting metastasis in 91% of patients. At resection, 50% were downstaged, 41% upstaged, and only 10% of patients had no change in final pathology. The investigators concluded that use of EUS did not predict lymph node metastasis accurately. A majority of these studies were conducted outside their facility, and the investigators suggested it was difficult to ascertain the quality of the EUS and whether adequate FNA was performed. It is evident that EUS may be a useful tool for assessing lymph nodes; however, best results are seen with the addition of FNA in experienced hands.

M Staging

Approximately 50% of patients present with advanced cancer, often with their presenting symptoms related to distant metastatic disease. The most commonly seen sites of distant involvement include liver, lung, bone, and peritoneal cavity. PET/CT (where a CT scan with IV contrast protocol is performed in conjunction with the PET scan) is the most accurate assessment of distant spread of tumor. CT scan alone provides suboptimal metastatic evaluation, with sensitivity of 91% and specificity of 52%. Diagnostic CT is valuable in the evaluation of structures, specifically the lung parenchyma, and can be critical when differentiating between pneumonia, pulmonary metastasis, tumor, and radiation-induced pulmonary fibrosis.

You and colleagues[15] examined the Ontario registry from 6 hospitals to determine if the use of PET/CT scan altered the clinical staging of esophageal cancer cases. From 2009 to 2011, 491 patient records were prospectively reviewed and followed for a median of 336 days. Conventional studies for staging included nuclear bone scan, brain imaging, CT scan, and, less frequently, EUS. PET/CT scan changed the stage of 118/491 patients (24%); 107 changed from M0 to M1, and 7 changed from M1b to M0. A total of 74/491 patients (15%) were upstaged from M1a to M1b. They showed a survival decline as the M stage increased. Although this study did not highlight which patients had confirmatory biopsy for the M disease, the investigators reported an approximately 3% false-positive rate. PET/CT scan is vital to establishing M disease and, when possible, biopsy of questionable avid lesions should be done to guide therapy.

Regarding the combined use of EUS, CT scan and PET scan in patients with locally advanced esophageal cancer, several studies have been done to determine what sequence is best for surgical planning. Schreurs and colleagues[10] studied the accuracy of staging using PET scan, CT scan, and EUS in esophageal cancer. A total of 216 operable patients underwent different staging strategies to evaluate which can best predict curative resectability. Tumor length was used as a benchmark to find a correlating staging regimen with the most accurate resectability assessment. Their results showed that a staging algorithm of PET scan followed by CT scan followed by EUS had the highest ratio of true-negative outcomes. When scenarios had EUS as the first staging modality, they had the least true-negative outcomes. The investigators concluded that EUS has the least to add to the surgeon's decision for resectability compared with PET and CT scans.

EUS can be reserved for cases of questionable resectability, and lymph node assessment may add to the clinical staging prior to surgical consideration. Because EUS has more interoperator variability compared with PET and CT scan, subjecting a patient to EUS scheduling may create delays in initiation of therapy. The best data of accuracy of EUS use come from high-volume centers, with studies showing lower-volume EUS centers have lower accuracy of detection. In patients with obstructing or near obstructing tumors, the value of EUS is reduced.[11] In such patients, having endoscopic confirmation of cancer followed by PET and CT scan may be the most optimal and expeditious pathway to their clinical staging.

Metastatic disease to the brain in esophageal cancer is less common than in other tumors. Routine brain imaging is not recommended by the NCCN staging guidelines.[1] Large studies looking at the incidence of distant brain metastasis failed to show a benefit in routine brain MRI staging for metastasis evaluation.[16]

The Memorial Sloan Kettering group[17] studied patients with locally advanced esophageal cancer who underwent trimodality treatment. A total of 1760 patients were analyzed, with a median follow-up of 4.58 years. At the end of the study, 686/1760 patients (39%) developed recurrence. By 5 years, isolated brain metastasis occurred in only 2.3% of patients, whereas 11% had locoregional and 27% had systemic disease. The median time to development of brain metastasis was approximately 1 year, with more than 80% of brain metastasis presenting within the first year postoperatively. A multivariate regression analysis found that only the presence of diabetes correlated with development of brain metastasis. The investigators suggest that following induction chemoradiation, brain imaging may be warranted in diabetic patients prior to their esophagectomy as part of their restaging. The authors advocate brain imaging in those with concerning neurologic symptoms. As an established alternative to brain MRI, evaluation for metastasis can be done with head CT scan.

RESTAGING FOLLOWING INDUCTION CHEMORADIATION

The Chemotherapy for Oesophageal Cancer Followed by Surgery Study (CROSS) trial demonstrated that overall survival is approximately doubled with trimodality therapy for squamous and adenocarcinoma of the esophagus.[18] Once a patient is identified as having a locally advanced tumor, a concurrent chemotherapy and radiotherapy regimen can be started. A restaging assessment generally is performed within 4 weeks of completion of therapy when induction-related inflammation decreases. The authors start with a history and physical, much like the initial evaluation to identify gross metastatic disease, as well as an evaluation of the patient's fitness for esophagectomy. Following clinical assessment, objective testing is required to restage the patient. PET/CT scan is the most accurate and reliable test available. Its largest pitfall may be its false-positive results. Diagnostic CT scan may be needed to differentiate between tumor or inflammation in surrounding lung parenchyma. Optimal timing for performing the restaging PET/CT is variable, with some centers advocating an early (2 weeks) post start of induction, whereas most centers wait until after induction therapy is complete. In the authors' practice, it is believed that a period of 4 weeks after conclusion of chemoradiation is appropriate. This time interval allows ongoing treatment effect after the conclusion date of chemoradiation and may decrease the rate of false-positive findings seen on PET/CT. In some cases, repeat imaging is delayed. For example, a patient may be too malnourished or rendered unfit to undergo an esophagectomy following chemoradiation. In such cases, that patient is reassessed clinically on a bimonthly basis. Once there is clinical improvement, the restaging PET/CT scan is obtained.

Swisher and colleagues[19] retrospectively analyzed 64 consecutive esophagectomy patients from 2001 to 2003. These patients all underwent trimodality therapy starting with chemoradiation then esophagectomy. Their protocol involved concurrent induction chemoradiation followed by restaging 4 weeks to 6 weeks after completion of therapy. Esophagectomy was performed 5 weeks to 8 weeks after completion of therapy. The endpoint was to identify which test correlated best with pathologic nonresponse to chemoradiation. Preinduction and postinduction CT scan width greater than 14.5 mm of tumor, EUS mucosal length greater than 1 cm, and PET SUV greater than 4 were used as markers to assess the specificity and sensitivity of each test. CT scan had sensitivity of 51% and a specificity of 69%. EUS had 56% sensitivity and 75% specificity. PET scan SUV had the best accuracy, with 62% sensitivity and 84% specificity. Survival at 18 months was 34% versus 77%, respectively, when an SUV less than 4 versus SUV 4 and above was used as a cutoff ($P = .01$). The investigators deduce that after chemoradiation, the nonviable tumor and fibrosis make EUS and CT scan less reliable tools to assess response. PET scan offers the best ability to capture viable tumor. Although it cannot rule out microscopic disease, it proves a vital addition in the decision to provide the patient with more induction therapy versus proceeding with esophagectomy. PET scan's ability to rule out progressive disease or new metastasis is unparalleled and is paramount prior to esophagectomy. Diagnostic CT scan still can be extremely useful as an adjunctive test to PET scan. It provides superior visualization of the lung parenchyma, which allows an astute surgeon the ability to differentiate between radiation-associated activity in the lungs, infection, and metastatic disease.

Staging laparoscopy also may have a role in some patients. The authors find it useful particularly in patients who require enteral nutrition due to bulky tumors. Staging laparoscopy can be used to identify peritoneal or liver metastasis; biopsy of suspicious intraabdominal radiographic findings as well as provide simultaneous feeding tube access.

Staging can be complex, with some studies becoming redundant based on subsequent studies or treatment decisions, all of which is made more difficult when they frequently are ordered by different physicians with different treatment plans. The authors' work-up remains relatively simple and is outlined in **Fig. 1**. Regardless of how a clinician proceeds, it is important to move expeditiously and consider scheduling tests in parallel with one another as opposed to in series to be most helpful.

STAGING IN THE FUTURE

Magnetic resonance imaging (MRI) is a mainstay for staging certain tumors, such as rectal cancer. Certain centers are using it as part of their staging algorithm for esophageal cancer.

Guo and colleagues[12] analyzed the use of MRI compared with CT/EUS in esophageal cancer patients in China. A total of 74 patients were enrolled to be staged either by MRI or by CT/EUS prior to their esophagectomy. Pathologic staging was compared between 2 staging modalities. Blinded readers to the scans were scored on sensitivity

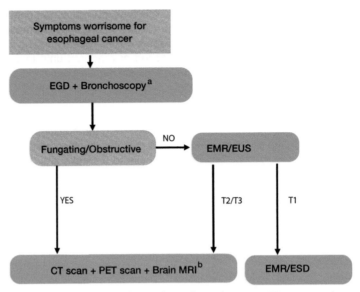

Fig. 1. Algorithm for staging work-up of esophageal cancer. CT, computed tomography; EGD, esophagogastroduodenoscopy; EMR, endoscopic mucosal resection; ESD, endoscopic submucosal dissection; EUS, endoscopic ultrasound; PET, positron emission tomography. [a]If tumor found at mid esophagus, should do bronchoscopic evaluation to evaluate for pulmonary involvement [b]Brain MRI can be done if neurological signs and symptoms present and suspicious of brain metastasis.

and specificity for each scan. For early cancers, MRI and EUS performed equally. For T3/T4 cancers, however, MRI had higher specificity (59% vs 93%; $P = .0015$). The same was seen for MRI versus CT scan. EUS and CT scan were comparable with respect to specificity. More than 75% of the patients had squamous cell carcinoma and had access to the rapid MRI scan used in this study. The investigators argue that this modality may be a useful addition to the esophageal cancer staging platform as it becomes more available.

Molecular testing for HER2-neu status, microsatellite instability status, programmed death ligand 1 expression, and NTRK gene fusions are reserved for management of advanced disease.[1] As understanding of tumor biology is expanded, future staging strategies incorporating these and other tests into the assessment of tumor spread may be seen.

Future studies are ongoing to analyze staging strategies and how they relate to survival following resection. The TIGER protocol is a multinational cohort study looking at the accuracy of staging using EUS, PET/CT, and endobronchial ultrasound in a standardized lymphadenectomy for esophagectomy patients.[20] The study is set to close accrual in 2021 and hopefully will add to the clinical assessment tools for this disease.

SUMMARY

Esophageal cancer spreads rapidly and still has one of the worst survival outcomes. Despite advances in multimodal therapy, survivorship data have not improved. Early staging and multidisciplinary discussion of the appropriate therapy needed are crucial to provide the best survival benefit. For early nonobstructing small lesions, EMR and

EUS can be used to stage early cancers and, at times, even provide definitive treatment. For fungating, near-obstructive lesions, PET/CT scan is required to assess for advanced disease and to rule out distant metastasis. For tumors near the level of the carina, additional evaluation with bronchoscopy of the airway is required to rule out T4 disease to the airway. For patients presenting with neurologic deficits, brain MRI can be done but is not a present recommendation. Following induction chemoradiotherapy for locally advanced disease, repeat PET/CT scan should be performed to assess tumor response to therapy. The authors hope the information provided in this article can help physicians as they choose their own staging plan, with a common goal of improving outcomes of this malignancy.

CLINICS CARE POINTS

- Endoscopic mucosal resection is an accurate staging tool for stage 1 esophageal cancer
- EUS is a useful adjunct for diagnosis of stage 2 esophageal cancer
- Locally advanced, fungating esophageal cancer often represents stage 3 esophageal cancer and efforts should be made to diagnose and initiate trimodality therapy promptly. Accurate staging can be accomplished efficiently with EGD PET/CT scans.
- Stage 4 esophageal cancer is assessed with PET scan. If neurologic symptoms are present, brain imaging with MRI or CT scan can be added to the evaluation.

DISCLOSURE

The authors have nothing to disclose.

REFERENCES

1. Available at: https://www.cancer.org/cancer/esophagus-cancer/detection-diagnosis-staging/survival-rates.html. Accessed October 14, 2020.
2. Amin MB, Edge SB, Greene FL. AJCC cancer staging manual. 8th edition. New York: Springer; 2017.
3. Brierley JD, Gospodarowicz MK, Wittekind CH. UICC TNM classification of malignant tumours. 8th edition. Sussex (UK): Wiley Blackwell; 2017.
4. Rice TW, Kelsen D, Blackstone EH, et al. Esophagus and esophagogastric junction. In: Amin MB, Edge SB, Greene FL, et al, editors. AJCC cancer staging Manual. 8th edition. New York: Springer; 2017. p. 185–202.
5. Ancona E, Rampado S, Cassaro M, et al. Prediction of lymph node status in superficial esophageal carcinoma. Ann Sur Oncol 2008;15(11):3278–88.
6. Hofstetter W. Treatment of clinical T2N0M0 esophageal cancer. Ann Surg Oncol 2014;21:3713–4.
7. Barbetta A, Schlottmann F, Nobel T, et al. Predictors of nodal metastases for clinical T2N0 esophageal adenocarcinoma. Ann Thorac Surg 2018;106(1):172–7.
8. Thosani N, Singh H, Kapadia A, et al. Diagnostic accuracy of EUS in differentiating mucosal versus submucosal invasion of superficial esophageal cancers: a systematic review and meta-analysis. Gastroinest Endosc 2012;75:242–53.
9. Shridhar R, Huston J, Meredith KL. Accuracy of Endoscopic Ultrasound Staging for T2N0 Esophageal Cancer: A National Cancer Database Analysis. J Gastrointest Oncol 2018;9(5):887–93.
10. Schreurs LMA, Janssens ACJW, Groen H, et al. Value of EUS in Determining Curative Resectability in Reference to CT and FDG-PET: The Optimal Sequence

in Preoperative Staging of Esophageal Cancer? Ann Surg Oncol 2016;23:1021–8. Available at: https://doi-org.elibrary.amc.edu/10.1245/s10434-011-1738-8.

11. Krill T, Baliss M, Roark R, et al. Accuracy of Endoscopic Ultrasound in Esophageal Cancer Staging. J Thorac Dis 2019;11:1609.

12. Guo J, Zhaoqi W, Qin J, et al. "A Prospective Analysis of the Diagnostic Accuracy of 3t MRI, CT and Endoscopic Ultrasound for Preoperative T Staging of Potentially Resectable Esophageal Cancer. Cancer Imaging 2020;20(1).

13. Cuellar SLB, Carter BW, Macapinlac HA, et al. Clinical staging of patients with early esophageal adenocarcinoma; dose FDG-PET/CT have a role? J Thorac Oncol 2014;9:1202–6.

14. Wang Y, Zhu L, Xia W, et al. Anatomy of lymphatic drainage of the esophagus and lymph node metastasis of thoracic esophageal cancer. Can Manag Res 2018;10: 6295–303.

15. You JJ, Wong RK, Darling G, et al. Clinical utility of 18F-fluorodeoxyglucose positron emission tomography/computed tomography in the staging of patients with potentially resectable esophageal cancer. J Thorac Oncol 2013;8:1563–9.

16. Wadhwa R, Taketa T, Correa A, et al. Incidence of brain metastases after trimodality therapy in patients with esophageal or gastroesophageal cancer: implications for screening and surveillance. Oncology 2013;85(4):204–7.

17. Nobel TB, Dave N, Eljalby M, et al. Incidence and risk factors for isolated esophageal cancer recurrence to the brain. Ann Thorac Surg 2020;109(2):329–36.

18. van Hagen P, Hulshof MC, van Lanschot JJ, et al. Preoperative chemoradiotherapy for esophageal or junctional cancer. N Engl J Med 2012;366:2074–84.

19. Swisher SG, Maish M, Erasmus JJ, et al. Utility of PET, CT, and EUS to identify pathology responders in esophageal cancer. Ann Thorac Surg 2004;78:1152–60.

20. Hagens ER, van Berge Henegouwen MI, van Sandick JW, et al. Distribution of lymph node metastasis in esophageal carcinoma [TIGER study]: study protocol of a multinational observational study. BMC Cancer 2019;19:662–70.

Recommendations for Surveillance and Management of Recurrent Esophageal Cancer Following Endoscopic Therapies

Chigozirim N. Ekeke, MD[a,1], Ernest G. Chan, MD, MPH[a,1],
Thomas Fabian, MD[b], Manuel Villa-Sanchez, MD[a],
James D. Luketich, MD[c,*]

KEYWORDS

- Esophageal malignancy • Minimally invasive esophagectomy
- Endoscopic treatment

KEY POINTS

- Endoscopic therapies for carefully selected, early-stage esophageal cancer can yield comparable oncologic results when compared with surgery.
- Careful patient selection and endoscopic surveillance are necessary to minimize the risk of recurrence.
- Multifocal disease occult nodal metastasis, positive margins, and evidence of lymphovascular invasion are some of the important risks associated with endoscopic resection failure.
- Endoscopic surveillance and follow-up imaging are necessary to detect any sign of recurrence or residual disease.
- Clinicians should make therapeutic recommendations based on the data not simply on their desire to avoid esophagectomy.

INTRODUCTION

The incidence of esophageal cancer has remained relatively stable over the last 20 years. In the United States and western countries, the prevalence of esophageal

[a] Department of Cardiothoracic Surgery, The University of Pittsburgh School of Medicine and the University of Pittsburgh Medical Center, 200 Lothrop Street, Suite C800, Pittsburgh, PA 15213, USA; [b] Department of Surgery, Section of Thoracic Surgery, Albany Medical Center, 43 New Scotland Avenue, MC-50, R-113, Albany, NY 12208, USA; [c] Department of Cardiothoracic Surgery, The University of Pittsburgh School of Medicine and the University of Pittsburgh Medical Center, 200 Lothrop Street, Suite C816, Pittsburgh, PA 15213, USA
[1] These authors contributed equally as co-first authors.
* Corresponding author.
E-mail address: luketichjd@upmc.edu

Surg Clin N Am 101 (2021) 415–426
https://doi.org/10.1016/j.suc.2021.03.004
0039-6109/21/© 2021 Elsevier Inc. All rights reserved.
surgical.theclinics.com

adenocarcinoma has surpassed squamous cell carcinoma (SCC). Although many patients present with advanced disease, with increased access to health care and endoscopy, more early-stage tumors are being found.[1,2]

With increased screening of Barrett patients, the percentage of patients diagnosed with early-stage tumors is 0.5%.[3] These patients may be managed either endoscopically or surgically, and these approaches were discussed in earlier articles. The interest in localized therapy is important, but it is important to keep in mind that nearly half of all patients with a new diagnosis of esophageal cancer already has systemic spread. Only 20% of patients is identified with early-stage disease, whereas another 35% to 40% of patients present with evidence of borderline resectable locoregional disease, that is, beyond endoscopic resection consideration.[4] Multimodal therapy has been shown to achieve the highest chance of curative success when significant locoregional nodal involvement exists. Therapeutic options may include chemotherapy alone, combined chemoradiation, or surgical resection. Despite poor survival at 5 years (19.9%),[5] it is important to identify patients with early-stage esophageal cancer and aggressively treat the disease and recognize when early endoscopic interventions will or will not work.[4] As surveillance protocols for Barrett disease continue to be refined and access to health care increases, the authors anticipate a higher number of esophageal neoplasms to be diagnosed at earlier stages.[6]

Currently, patients have several therapeutic options depending on the extent of their disease, comorbidities, and overall performance metrics. Endoscopic intervention has an acceptable safety profile and minimal risk and has become a widely adopted alternative approach for treating premalignant and early, esophageal neoplasms in well-selected patients. Esophagectomy remains a viable treatment option even for those with early-stage esophageal cancer and remains the gold standard by which to compare less-invasive procedures. In some centers, surgical resection remains the treatment of choice, for example, young and fit patients who may otherwise have a significant lifetime risk of recurrence if only endoscopic mucosal resection (EMR) is performed.[7] At the authors' institution, once a stage Ib is diagnosed, they recommend performing a minimally invasive esophagectomy, given the significant risk of locoregional lymph node involvement (15%–27%).[7–9] Despite the ongoing developments in endoscopic intervention, managing locally recurrent disease and the need for long-term surveillance make minimally invasive esophagectomy (MIE) preferable in many patients even though they may be candidates for endoscopic therapy. Reported recurrence rates of esophageal cancer following endoscopic therapies range from 3% to 32%.[10–12]

The report by Ells and colleagues[7] of a long-term complete remission (CR) rate of 96% over a 57-month follow-up period in patients with early-stage esophageal cancer treated with endoscopic resection is encouraging. However, it is important to note that this was a highly selected group of early-stage patients, and of the 1718 patients in this report that were referred for endoscopic resection, more than 40% were excluded because of unfavorable criteria, such as deeper invasion beyond a T1a, or other unfavorable criteria. In addition to endoscopic resection, in the favorable group, the majority underwent some form of ablative therapy, such as argon beam coagulation, radiofrequency ablation (RFA), or phototherapy. Other important details one must consider before deciding to reject esophagectomy is that these results are from a highly specialized center with very meticulous follow-up in terms of biopsies, endoscopic ultrasound (EUS), and pathologic assessment. This level of expertise is not widely available.

In the following pages, the authors describe in more detail the treatment of early-stage esophageal cancer, patterns of recurrent esophageal cancer, surveillance, and management of recurrent esophageal cancer following endoscopic treatment options.

INDICATIONS FOR ENDOSCOPIC TREATMENT OF EARLY-STAGE ESOPHAGEAL CANCER

Intraepithelial Neoplasia (Dysplasia)

In the most recent iteration of the National Comprehensive Cancer Network (NCCN) Esophageal and Esophagogastric Junction Cancers Guidelines 2020, major changes include the rebranding of high-grade dysplasia (HGD; previously carcinoma in situ) in Barrett esophagus as intraepithelial neoplasia or Tis.[13] Current recommendations for treatment of esophageal intraepithelial neoplasia include endoscopic treatment. Adjunct ablations may be required to ensure adequate treatment of the lesion.

Early-Stage Esophageal Cancer

Based on the American Joint Committee on Cancer 8th Edition Staging System for esophageal cancer, early-stage esophageal malignancy staged as T1 disease is defined as a neoplastic lesion of esophageal origin that is limited to the lamina propria, muscular mucosa, or submucosa.[14] Within this T category, the disease is further differentiated into T1a (tumor invading into the lamina propria or muscularis mucosae) and T1b (tumor invading the submucosa). This differentiation is important, as it pertains to the threshold for endoscopic therapies versus surgery, while considering risk of disease progression. Angiolymphatic invasion (ALI) is rarely evident (0%–2% lymph node metastasis in T1a) with mucosal involvement, but submucosal lesions (T1b) portend to higher risk for ALI and poorly differentiation grade with a risk of lymph node involving being reported between 13% and 44%.[7–9] Along with ALI, poor differentiation grade, the presence of increased depth of invasion, and tumor diameter greater than 2 cm are risk factors for lymphatic spread. The submucosal layer is known for its abundant lymphatic channels, which can be a predilection for distant dissemination. These features are risk factors for failure after endoscopic treatment.

Accurate EUS staging of T1a is 85% sensitivity and 87% specificity, whereas sensitivity and specificity in T1b disease are 86%.[15] Computed tomography (CT) and fluorodeoxyglucose-PET scans have poor sensitivity (50%–57%) for celiac lymph node metastases, thus are useful primarily for diagnosing distant metastases.[15] Currently, endoscopic resection is only recommended for T1a disease and select cases for T1b disease.[16] There is a distinct difference between adenocarcinomas and squamous carcinoma of the esophagus and their propensity for lymph node metastasis. Per NCCN guidelines, while patients with T1b adenocarcinoma of the esophagus can be carefully selected to undergo EMR, patients with T1b squamous cell of the esophagus should not because of the higher risk of nodal metastasis associated with the squamous cell histology.[13] Nonetheless, this approach allows for the potential of curative resection, while assessing pathologic depth of invasion, to accurately determine the true T stage with pathologic confirmation. At the authors' institution, they commonly use EMR for T1a disease. Some centers have advocated endoscopic submucosal dissection (ESD) for deeper or more extensive surface lesions, but this is not available in many centers. Multifocal disease, occult nodal metastasis, and evidence of lymphovascular invasion (LVI) are risks associated with endoscopic therapy failure for early-stage esophageal cancers.[17,18] Therefore, the authors recommend a careful and complete work-up with expert pathologic assessment of the EMR specimen, and the EUS findings before embarking on any endoscopic resection strategy as the best choice for early-stage esophageal cancers.

Factors associated with increased failures in patients undergoing endoscopic tumor therapy

1. Lymphovascular invasion

2. T1b-submucosal involvement

3. Squamous cell carcinoma

4. Deep lesions

5. Piecemeal resection

6. Lesions >2 cm

BENEFITS OF ENDOSCOPIC THERAPIES FOR EARLY-STAGE ESOPHAGEAL CANCER

Endoscopic therapies, such as EMR and ESD, with associated ablative therapies, such as argon beam, photodynamic therapy, and RFA are associated with less morbidity in comparison to esophagectomy.[19] The decision tree always includes expert evaluation of the EMR specimen, which provides an extensive tissue sample for accurate pathologic staging. Therefore, EMR can be used for accurate assessment and staging as well as therapeutic procedure. Appropriate use of EMR allows for identification of risk factors as described above. These risk factors for failure in turn assist the clinician and patient to determine the most appropriate treatment. In addition to EMR, endoscopic ablative therapies may serve as adjunct tools to endoscopic removal and treats any residual dysplastic lesions in the presence of Barrett's esophagus (BE) and early-stage disease. photodynamic therapy (PDT), argon beam laser coagulation, cryotherapy, and radiofrequency all have been used for ablating residual dysplastic mucosa after endoscopic resection.[19,20]

Overall, successful eradication of T1a malignancy with the use of EMR has been reported to be more than 95%.[7,21] Multiple Japanese studies highlighted successful resection (100%) and 80% cure rate for T1b following utilization of ESD.[22,23] The benefit of reduced morbidity (1%–3%), mortality risk (0%–1%),[15] and organ preservation with the endoscopic approach compares favorably with esophagectomy (morbidity: 20%–50%, mortality: 2%–5%)[24–27] for early-stage disease. Although these results are overall very impressive, it is important to note that these results can differ when stratifying by histology. For example, patients with squamous cell histology have a higher risk of nodal metastasis despite being an early-stage cancer. This finding is especially highlighted in patients with SCC of the esophagus that has invaded the muscularis mucosal layers (M3), with reported incidence of nodal metastasis as high as 11.8%.[28]

PATTERNS OF RECURRENCE AFTER ENDOSCOPIC TREATMENT

Recurrence rates for endoscopic treatment of early-stage esophageal cancer may be as high as 21%.[29] Manner and colleagues[7] retrospectively analyzed endoscopic remission rates in 66 patients with T1a disease. In their series, 87% (n = 53) of the patients achieved CR following endoscopic therapy, but 97% CR was observed in patients with lesions less than 2 cm. Endoscopic therapy included endoscopic resection along with use of ablative adjuncts (argon, RFA, and PDT) in areas of residual Barrett disease. Metachronous lesions were observed in 10 of 53 patients, and 84% (n = 51) achieved long-term remission.[7] Pech and colleagues[30] documented a 22%

rate of recurrent and metachronous lesions following endoscopic resection. A separate retrospective study from South Korea identified risk factors for metachronous recurrence following esophageal ESD in 253 patients with T1a SCC.[31] In this study, the surgeons used Lugol chromoendoscopy before ESD to assess targeted lesion appearance.[31] A univariate and multivariate analyses revealed multiple Lugol-void lesions (LVL), margins of the main LVL, and tumor differentiation were risk factors for metachronous malignancy following endoscopic treatment. Other risk factors for metachronous lesions following endoscopic treatment include extensive or residual dysplastic Barrett disease, and multifocal neoplastic lesions.[30–33] Furthermore, the duplication of muscularis mucosa may be indicative of aggressive disease, despite its intramucosal location. A multi-institutional study evaluated 50 patients with HGD or T1a disease.[34] In this study, 46 patients (92%) showed evidence of esophageal cancer that was limited to the muscularis mucosa. ALI and nodal metastasis were evident in 17% and 10%, respectively, further indicating the challenge in staging superficial adenocarcinomas.[34]

Given the multiple risks, careful surveillance after treatment is required. A separate retrospective analysis assessed the outcomes of patients that underwent EMR (n = 23) and esophagectomy (n = 49) for T1b esophageal adenocarcinoma.[35] Within 3 years, 23% of patients (n = 5) had evidence of local recurrence versus 4.7% (n = 1), respectively, and of those, 3 (13%) experienced regional and distal recurrence. Patients with ALI, tumors greater than 2 cm, and poorly differentiated lesions were at higher risk of nodal metastasis and increased risk for distant recurrence following EMR. Furthermore, in patients with low-risk features (no ALI, <2 cm lesion, well to moderate differentiation), EMR for T1b disease had a higher risk of local recurrence in comparison to esophagectomy. In the same study, many of these local recurrences were salvaged with either repeat EMR (n = 2) or esophagectomy (n = 1).[35] **Table 1** provides a brief multistudy summary of the rate of recurrence following endoscopic resection for early-stage esophageal cancer.

SURVEILLANCE FOR RECURRENCE FOLLOWING ENDOSCOPIC THERAPIES

Presently, NCCN guidelines regarding surveillance after endoscopic therapy fall under 3 groups: patients with completely resected malignancy, persistent Barrett's or dysplasia. Recommendations in this group state endoscopic assessment with biopsy should be performed at or greater than 6 weeks or if there is suspicion for disease recurrence.[13] During endoscopic surveillance, careful attention to detail for mucosal surface changes is recommended along with multiple biopsies of any visualized

Table 1
Recurrent disease following endoscopic resection

Study	Number of Patients	Complete Resection (%)	Recurrence Rate (%)
Shimizu et al,[48] 2001	82	100	14.6 at 5 y
Nomura et al,[37] 2000	51	100	8 at 6 y
Pech et al[49] 2004	29	92	16.7 at 4 y
Katada et al,[50] 2005	116	100	20 at 3 y
Fujishiro et al,[51] 2006	43	100	2.3 at 6 mo
Kim et al,[31] 2020	253	84	8.3 at 9 y
Nelson et al,[32] 2018	23	n/a	39 at 3 y

Abbvreviation: n/a, not applicable.

abnormal appearing mucosa. Furthermore, surgeons and endoscopists should note any subtle dysplastic mucosal changes, strictures, and any gross changes from previous endoscopic examination. Beyond that, NCCN guidelines separate tumors into 2 more categories, Tis/T1a or T1b tumors. In Tis/T1a, recommendations are endoscopy every 3 months for the first year, and endoscopy every 6 months for the second year, and then annually. No imaging surveillance is recommended in this group.

In T1b, recommendations are EMR-treated patients, endoscopy every 3 months for first year, endoscopy every 4 to 6 months for the second year, and then annually. Imaging may be considered every 12 months for up to 3 years. The NCCN also states that EUS as part of surveillance endoscopy may be considered as an adjunct to endoscopy.

At the authors' institution, their surveillance recommendations are determined by histopathologic results of the first endoscopic resection. Specifically, patients are separated into low- and high-risk groups based on T stage, size, and presence of LVI. The low-risk group includes T = Tis or T1a, less than 2 cm and with no evidence of LVI, versus a second group that includes patients with either ≥T1b or >2 cm, or that have LVI.

In the first group, the authors believe patients should undergo upper gastrointestinal endoscopy every 3 months for the first year, every 6 months for the second year, and then annually indefinitely. Imaging is not recommended as a surveillance tool in these patients although it may be performed as part of staging. These patients should also undergo treatment for any other areas of Barrett, and this should coincide with the surveillance endoscopies.

For patients, in the high-risk group whereby risk of failure includes local, regional, and distant recurrence, surveillance is different. These patients would routinely be staged before treatment with a PET scan. In some cases, the EMR may precede the PET scan, and the authors believe it remains an important part of staging patients, particularly T1b tumors and higher. Serial endoscopy is recommended as described in the first group of patients, every 3 months for the first year, every 6 months for the second year, and then annually indefinitely. The authors also perform a CT every 4 to 6 months for the first 2 years and then annually indefinitely to monitor for any signs of distant recurrence. No data exist to support surveillance with PET scan. It is considered unnecessary in T1a tumors. Antidotally, some have argued a limited role of a PET scan as a single interval scan perhaps 6 to 12 months after treatment for 1B tumors to rule out regional lymph node recurrence; no evidence at present supports this approach.

Low-risk tumor surveillance

Esophagoscopy

Every 3 months—1 year

Every 6 months—1 year

Every year– lifetime

High-risk tumor surveillance.

Esophagoscopy

Every 3 months—1 year

Every 4-6 months—1 year

Every year—lifetime

CT scan
Every 3 months—1 year
Every 6 months—1 year
Every year—lifetime

In the event any abnormalities are identified, reevaluation with repeat EMR or EUS has been found to have a high sensitivity upward of 95% for recurrent disease.[36] Imaging may be warranted to evaluate these changes; the authors do not routinely add or recommend EUS in the absence of abnormal findings.

OPTIONS FOR FAILED ENDOSCOPIC TREATMENTS AND THEIR OUTCOMES
Endoscopic Treatment

With proper surveillance, failures will be identified. Recurrences may be local, regional, or distant. For patients with local recurrence, successful repeat endoscopic therapy for recurrent has been reported.[30,37]

Reevaluation of these tumors with EUS or repeat EMR is appropriate. At University of Pittsburgh Medical Center, recurrent T1a disease in the setting of a patient who is fit for surgical resection, the authors will recommend esophagectomy for definitive therapy. If the patient is deemed too high risk for surgical resection, they will recommend a repeat attempt at EMR. Other institutions advocate for repeat EMR despite prior failures, and this can be a successful approach.

Pech's series reported an 85% success rate in patients that experienced recurrence of HGD or intramucosal carcinoma (14.5% recurrence rate) following index endoscopic treatment. Techniques to reduce this risk include RFA, ESD, and circumferential endoscopic resection of high-risk Barrett mucosa and have been introduced to prevent recurrence after initial malignancy eradication with endoscopic technique.[38] Nomuru and colleagues[37] conducted a retrospective study (n = 51) that assessed patient characteristics and outcomes following endoscopic resection in patients with T1 esophageal malignancy. Three patients underwent treatment for recurrence. Two patients were treated successfully with repeat EMR, whereas local recurrence arose in the patient that received only radiation treatment for the initial recurrence.[37] Nelson and colleagues[35] reported patients (n = 5) presenting with local recurrence following EMR for T1b disease; 2 patients underwent repeat EMR. The remaining patients underwent surgical resection (n = 1) or radiation (n = 2).[35]

Surgical Treatment

Currently, the authors' institution recommends esophagectomy for patients that present with index T1b or recurrent esophageal malignancy following failed endoscopic therapy. Surgical options may include MIE, robotic-assisted esophagectomy, transthoracic (Ivor Lewis), transhiatal esophagectomy, or 3-incision modified McKeown esophagectomy.[39] Resection approaches are dependent on location of the recurrence and surgeon preference. Despite the known morbidity and mortality risk of esophagectomy, the authors' group has successfully adopted the minimally invasive approach. In their retrospective study of 1033 patients, the median length of stay in the intensive care unit and overall length of stay in the hospital was 2 and 8 days, respectively. Thirty-day operative mortality was less than 2%.[40] More than 10% of patients had stage I esophageal malignancy in the authors' study. Hunt and colleagues[17] reported outcomes in 15 patients who underwent esophagectomy at a mean time of 13 months after a mean number of 4.1 failed endotherapies (EMR and RFA). Of these, 15 patients 3

(20%) were found to have node-positive disease. This finding suggests that either the patients were inappropriately selected for esophageal preservation or progressed while undergoing failed EMRs.[17] No recurrence was observed at a mean follow-up time of 20 months after esophagectomy. A separate multi-institutional study (7 major centers) from Molena and colleagues[41] reported surgical outcomes of 23 patients with submucosal esophageal adenocarcinoma. These patients underwent esophagectomy at a median of 2 months after endoscopic resection. Of the patients, 26% (n = 6) were found to have positive nodal disease. At a median follow-up time of 37 months, 91% of patients were alive and had no evidence of residual or recurrent disease. Disease-specific 5-year survival was reported to be 67% in patients with pathologic-confirmed nodal disease and 100% in patients with N0 disease at the time of esophagectomy. Both Molena and Hunt demonstrate the most dreaded of all complications, which is undertreatment of tumor.[17,41] Although data show that some of these patients can be salvaged with resection, not all will be. Furthermore, these recurrences and then treatment were performed in the setting of academic institutions and clinical studies. It is likely that outside of that clinical format recurrences will not be identified as early and lead to even more undertreatment of curable esophageal cancer.

Dickinson and colleagues used an EMR histology-based risk-scoring tool, in a cohort of 51 patients with clinical T1 esophageal adenocarcinoma. This risk-scoring tool stratified a patient's risk of lymph node metastasis based on tumor size, differentiation, depth, and LVI once diagnosed with T1 esophageal adenocarcinoma (**Table 2**).[42] Based on this risk scoring tool, patients were deemed low predicted risk of lymph node metastasis ($\leq$2%) if they scored 0 to 1 points, moderate risk (3%–6% predicted risk of lymph node metastasis) if they scored between 2 and 4 points, and high risk ($\geq$7% predicted risk of lymph node metastasis) if they scored 5 or more. Development of this tool found that LVI and tumor size were the strongest predictors of lymph node involvement in these patients. With this tool, they found that 27% of patients were upstaged after undergoing esophagectomy. Of the 51 patients, 10 patients (19.6%) were found to have nodal involvement, 7 of which were deemed high risk based on their scoring tool.[43]

Esophagectomy for acute and nonacute failure of ESD is appropriate and can be successful. Wang and colleagues[44] describes 32 patients that underwent esophagectomy after ESD. Indications for esophagectomy following ESD included disease recurrence, esophageal stricture, or residual tumor at the ESD specimen margin, and perforation. There was 0% in-hospital mortality 30 days after esophagectomy. Complete resection

Table 2
Tool for predicting lymph node metastasis in patients with T1 esophageal adenocarcinoma

Variable	Point System[a]	
Tumor size	Value is dependent on tumor size per centimeter	+1 per cm (microscopic disease = +0)
Depth	T1a	+0
	T1b	+2
Differentiation	Well	+0
	Moderate	+3
	Poor	+3
Lymphovascular invasion	Presence of lymphovascular invasion on histology	+6

[a] Predictive risk for lymph node metastasis: low risk, 0 to 1 points; moderate risk, 2 to 4 points; high risk, $\geq$5 points.

was achieved in all patients. The recommended period between ESD and elective surgical resection was 30 days to allow for resolution of esophageal edema.[44]

SUMMARY/FUTURE DIRECTIONS

Endoscopic resection is an accepted approach for treating HGD and node-negative–early-stage esophageal cancer in select groups of patients. Excellent results with EMR have been well described, and the 30-day mortality (<1%) is favorable, but with the advent of centers of excellence performing minimally invasive and robot-assisted esophagectomy, mortalities of just less than 1% have also been reported; thus, mortality is not the main issue any longer.[45,46] Although the authors acknowledge the morbidity of MIE and the potential for negative quality-of-life impact, several groups, including the authors', have reported excellent quality-of-life scores after successful MIE.[47] Despite the high success rate for tumor eradication with EMR, studies still report a recurrence rate as high as 32%.[10-12] Endoscopists and surgeons must remember these favorable endoscopic resection reports are from very high-volume centers with excellent endoscopists, high-tech endoscopic ultrasound, and expert pathologists, all of which are not available in most medical centers. In addition, there is the inherent disadvantage of limited lymph node assessment and inability to remove involved nodes that are positive in up to 26% of patients.[41] Endoscopic experience and aggressive surgical approach for failed therapy are necessary to successfully treat early-stage esophageal malignancy. Favorable outcomes following surgical resection for failed endoscopic therapy have been reported[44] but are not ideal. Clinicians would be well advised to make therapeutic recommendations based on the data not simply on their desire to avoid esophagectomy. In discussions with patients, the shortcomings and challenges of all treatments should be pointed out so that ultimately the patient is satisfied with their choices.

CLINICS CARE POINTS

- Endoscopic mucosal resection is first-line intervention for accurate and definitive diagnosis of high-grade dysplasia and T1a esophageal malignancy.

- Postendoscopic surveillance should include repeat endoscopic visualization and possible adjunct ablative therapy for residual high-grade dysplasia or Barrett disease based on pathologic assessment of the resected specimen and surrounding random and directed biopsies.

- Risk factors for recurrent esophageal malignancy following endoscopic treatment include piecemeal endoscopic mucosal resection, lymphatic invasion, extended segmental Barrett disease, residual dysplastic Barrett esophagus after remission, no ablative therapy of Barrett esophagus after resection, multifocal neoplastic lesions, and complete response greater than 10 months.

- Surveillance following endoscopic treatment of early-stage esophageal malignancy should include repeat esophagogastroduodenoscopy every 3 to 6 months (first 1–2 years), every 6 to 12 months (3–5 years), and annually (>5 years). More favorable biopsies during surveillance may lessen the number of endoscopies, but as discussed, the presence of dysplasia and other pathologic features may increase this need.

- Evidence of recurrent disease or residual disease after endoscopic therapy should be treated with minimally invasive or robotic esophagectomy unless the patient is high risk, in which repeat endoscopic mucosal resection should be considered (with the possibility of ablation therapy and addition of chemoradiation for more extensive recurrences).

DISCLOSURE

The authors have nothing to disclose.

REFERENCES

1. Pennathur A, Farkas A, Krasinskas AM, et al. Esophagectomy for T1 esophageal cancer: outcomes in 100 patients and implications for endoscopic therapy. Ann Thorac Surg 2009;87(4):1048–54 [discussion 54-5].
2. Polednak AP. Trends in survival for both histologic types of esophageal cancer in US surveillance, epidemiology and end results areas. Int J Cancer 2003;105(1): 98–100.
3. Kroep S, Lansdorp-Vogelaar I, Rubenstein JH, et al. An accurate cancer incidence in Barrett's esophagus: a best estimate using published data and modeling. Gastroenterology 2015;149(3):577–85.e4 [quiz e14-5].
4. Higuchi K, Koizumi W, Tanabe S, et al. Current management of esophageal squamous-cell carcinoma in Japan and other countries. Gastrointest Cancer Res 2009;3(4):153–61.
5. Siegel RL, Miller KD, Jemal A. Cancer statistics, 2020. CA Cancer J Clin 2020; 70(1):7–30.
6. Choi SE, Hur C. Screening and surveillance for Barrett's esophagus: current issues and future directions. Curr Opin Gastroenterol 2012;28(4):377–81.
7. Manner H, Pech O, Heldmann Y, et al. Efficacy, safety, and long-term results of endoscopic treatment for early stage adenocarcinoma of the esophagus with low-risk sm1 invasion. Clin Gastroenterol Hepatol 2013;11(6):630–5 [quiz e45].
8. Stein HJ, Feith M, Bruecher BLDM, et al. Early esophageal cancer: pattern of lymphatic spread and prognostic factors for long-term survival after surgical resection. Ann Surg 2005;242(4):566–75.
9. Ballard DD, Choksi N, Lin J, et al. Outcomes of submucosal (T1b) esophageal adenocarcinomas removed by endoscopic mucosal resection. World J Gastrointest Endosc 2016;8(20):763–9.
10. Nakagawa K, Koike T, Iijima K, et al. Comparison of the long-term outcomes of endoscopic resection for superficial squamous cell carcinoma and adenocarcinoma of the esophagus in Japan. Am J Gastroenterol 2014;109(3):348–56.
11. Saligram S, Chennat J, Hu H, et al. Endotherapy for superficial adenocarcinoma of the esophagus: an American experience. Gastrointest Endosc 2013;77(6): 872–6.
12. Yamashina T, Ishihara R, Nagai K, et al. Long-term outcome and metastatic risk after endoscopic resection of superficial esophageal squamous cell carcinoma. Am J Gastroenterol 2013;108(4):544–51.
13. Network NCC. NCCN clinical practice guidelines in oncology (NCCN guidelines): esophageal and esophagogastric junction cancers. Version 4.2020 2020.
14. Rice TW, Patil DT, Blackstone EH. AJCC/UICC staging of cancers of the esophagus and esophagogastric junction: application to clinical practice. Ann Cardiothorac Surg 2017;6(2):119.
15. Patel V, Burbridge RA. Endoscopic approaches for early-stage esophageal cancer: current options. Curr Oncol Rep 2015;17(1):421.
16. Rice TW, Blackstone EH, Goldblum JR, et al. Superficial adenocarcinoma of the esophagus. J Thorac Cardiovasc Surg 2001;122(6):1077–90.
17. Hunt BM, Louie BE, Schembre DB, et al. Outcomes in patients who have failed endoscopic therapy for dysplastic Barrett's metaplasia or early esophageal cancer. Ann Thorac Surg 2013;95(5):1734–40.

18. Altorki NK, Lee PC, Liss Y, et al. Multifocal neoplasia and nodal metastases in T1 esophageal carcinoma: implications for endoscopic treatment. Ann Surg 2008; 247(3):434–9.

19. Pacifico RJ, Wang KK, Wongkeesong LM, et al. Combined endoscopic mucosal resection and photodynamic therapy versus esophagectomy for management of early adenocarcinoma in Barrett's esophagus. Clin Gastroenterol Hepatol 2003; 1(4):252–7.

20. Dumot JA, Vargo JJ 2nd, Falk GW, et al. An open-label, prospective trial of cryo-spray ablation for Barrett's esophagus high-grade dysplasia and early esophageal cancer in high-risk patients. Gastrointest Endosc 2009;70(4):635–44.

21. Ciocirlan M, Lapalus MG, Hervieu V, et al. Endoscopic mucosal resection for squamous premalignant and early malignant lesions of the esophagus. Endoscopy 2007;39(1):24–9.

22. Ono S, Fujishiro M, Niimi K, et al. Long-term outcomes of endoscopic submucosal dissection for superficial esophageal squamous cell neoplasms. Gastrointest Endosc 2009;70(5):860–6.

23. Takahashi H, Arimura Y, Masao H, et al. Endoscopic submucosal dissection is superior to conventional endoscopic resection as a curative treatment for early squamous cell carcinoma of the esophagus (with video). Gastrointest Endosc 2010;72(2):255–64, 64.e1-2.

24. Hölscher AH, Bollschweiler E, Schneider PM, et al. Early adenocarcinoma in Barrett's oesophagus. Br J Surg 1997;84(10):1470–3.

25. Thomas P, Doddoli C, Neville P, et al. Esophageal cancer resection in the elderly. Eur J Cardiothorac Surg 1996;10(11):941–6.

26. Chang AC, Ji H, Birkmeyer NJ, et al. Outcomes after transhiatal and transthoracic esophagectomy for cancer. Ann Thorac Surg 2008;85(2):424–9.

27. Raymond DP, Seder CW, Wright CD, et al. Predictors of major morbidity or mortality after resection for esophageal cancer: a Society of Thoracic Surgeons general thoracic surgery database risk adjustment model. Ann Thorac Surg 2016; 102(1):207–14.

28. Li B, Chen H, Xiang J, et al. Prevalence of lymph node metastases in superficial esophageal squamous cell carcinoma. J Thorac Cardiovasc Surg 2013;146(5): 1198–203.

29. Pech O, May A, Rabenstein T, et al. Endoscopic resection of early oesophageal cancer. Gut 2007;56(11):1625–34.

30. Pech O, Behrens A, May A, et al. Long-term results and risk factor analysis for recurrence after curative endoscopic therapy in 349 patients with high-grade intraepithelial neoplasia and mucosal adenocarcinoma in Barrett's oesophagus. Gut 2008;57(9):1200–6.

31. Kim GH, Min YW, Lee H, et al. Risk factors of metachronous recurrence after endoscopic submucosal dissection for superficial esophageal squamous cell carcinoma. PLoS One 2020;15(9):e0238113.

32. Lahmann PH, Pandeya N, Webb PM, et al. Body mass index, long-term weight change, and esophageal squamous cell carcinoma: is the inverse association modified by smoking status? Cancer 2012;118(7):1901–9.

33. Prasad GA, Wu TT, Wigle DA, et al. Endoscopic and surgical treatment of mucosal (T1a) esophageal adenocarcinoma in Barrett's esophagus. Gastroenterology 2009;137(3):815–23.

34. Abraham SC, Krasinskas AM, Correa AM, et al. Duplication of the muscularis mucosae in Barrett esophagus: an underrecognized feature and its implication for staging of adenocarcinoma. Am J Surg Pathol 2007;31(11):1719–25.

35. Nelson DB, Dhupar R, Katkhuda R, et al. Outcomes after endoscopic mucosal resection or esophagectomy for submucosal esophageal adenocarcinoma. J Thorac Cardiovasc Surg 2018;156(1):406–13.e3.
36. Lightdale CJ, Botet JF, Kelsen DP, et al. Diagnosis of recurrent upper gastrointestinal cancer at the surgical anastomosis by endoscopic ultrasound. Gastrointest Endosc 1989;35(5):407–12.
37. Nomura T, Boku N, Ohtsu A, et al. Recurrence after endoscopic mucosal resection for superficial esophageal cancer. Endoscopy 2000;32(4):277–80.
38. Seewald S, Akaraviputh T, Seitz U, et al. Circumferential EMR and complete removal of Barrett's epithelium: a new approach to management of Barrett's esophagus containing high-grade intraepithelial neoplasia and intramucosal carcinoma. Gastrointest Endosc 2003;57(7):854–9.
39. Pennathur A, Gibson MK, Jobe BA, et al. Oesophageal carcinoma. Lancet 2013; 381(9864):400–12.
40. Luketich JD, Pennathur A, Awais O, et al. Outcomes after minimally invasive esophagectomy: review of over 1000 patients. Ann Surg 2012;256(1):95–103.
41. Molena D, Schlottmann F, Boys JA, et al. Esophagectomy following endoscopic resection of submucosal esophageal cancer: a highly curative procedure even with nodal metastases. J Gastrointest Surg 2017;21(1):62–7.
42. Lee L, Ronellenfitsch U, Hofstetter WL, et al. Predicting lymph node metastases in early esophageal adenocarcinoma using a simple scoring system. J Am Coll Surg 2013;217(2):191–9.
43. Dickinson KJ, Wang K, Zhang L, et al. Esophagectomy outcomes in the endoscopic mucosal resection era. Ann Thorac Surg 2017;103(3):890–7.
44. Wang W-P, Ni P-Z, Yang J-L, et al. Esophagectomy after endoscopic submucosal dissection for esophageal carcinoma. J Thorac Dis 2018;10(6):3253–61.
45. Lv L, Hu W, Ren Y, et al. Minimally invasive esophagectomy versus open esophagectomy for esophageal cancer: a meta-analysis. Onco Targets Ther 2016;9: 6751–62.
46. Yang Y, Zhang X, Li B, et al. Robot-assisted esophagectomy (RAE) versus conventional minimally invasive esophagectomy (MIE) for resectable esophageal squamous cell carcinoma: protocol for a multicenter prospective randomized controlled trial (RAMIE trial, robot-assisted minimally invasive esophagectomy). BMC Cancer 2019;19(1):608.
47. Pennathur A, Awais O, Luketich JD. Minimally invasive esophagectomy for Barrett's with high-grade dysplasia and early adenocarcinoma of the esophagus. J Gastrointest Surg 2010;14(6):948–50.
48. Shimizu Y, Tukagoshi H, Fujita M, et al. Metachronous squamous cell carcinoma of the esophagus arising after endoscopic mucosal resection. Gastrointest Endosc 2001;54(2):190–4.
49. Pech O, Gossner L, May A, et al. Endoscopic resection of superficial esophageal squamous-cell carcinomas: Western experience. Am J Gastroenterol 2004;99(7): 1226–32.
50. Katada C, Muto M, Manabe T, et al. Local recurrence of squamous-cell carcinoma of the esophagus after EMR. Gastrointest Endosc 2005;61(2):219–25.
51. Fujishiro M, Yahagi N, Kakushima N, et al. Endoscopic submucosal dissection of esophageal squamous cell neoplasms. Clin Gastroenterol Hepatol 2006;4(6): 688–94.

Surgical Management of Early Esophageal Cancer

Facundo Iriarte, MD, Stacey Su, MD, Roman V. Petrov, MD, PhD,
Charles T. Bakhos, MD, MS, Abbas E. Abbas, MD, MS*

KEYWORDS

- Early esophageal cancer • Esophagectomy • Robotic-assisted esophagectomy
- RAMIE

KEY POINTS

- Except in very superficial tumors, the standard of care for early esophageal cancer is esophagectomy.
- Minimally invasive approaches are being used for esophageal cancer treatment
- Robotic esophagectomy has several technical advantages in the treatment of early esophageal cancer.

 Video content accompanies this article at http://www.interventional.theclinics. com.

INTRODUCTION

Over the past 50 years, few cancers have seen as dramatic a rise in incidence as esophageal cancer. The number of new cases has risen from just 0.5 per 100,000 person-years in the 1970s to approximately 4.2 per 100,000 person-years.[1] Unfortunately, this has not been matched with as dramatic an improvement in outcomes. The number of new deaths from esophageal cancer is almost the same as that of new cases.[2,3] Based on the Surveillance, Epidemiology, and End Results database, it is estimated that only 30% of tumors at presentation are early or limited to the primary site whereas more than 70% of patients have regional (31%) or distant (38%) disease at the time of diagnosis. This is pertinent especially because the mortality rate from this disease rises dramatically with increased stage.[3,4] It, therefore, is of paramount importance to attempt to aggressively diagnose and treat this disease in its early stages.

This article discusses the management of early esophageal cancer (EEC) with special emphasis on the technical details of robotic esophagectomy for adenocarcinoma

Division of Thoracic Surgery, Department of Thoracic Medicine and Surgery, Temple University Hospital and Fox Chase Comprehensive Cancer Center, Philadelphia, PA, USA
* Corresponding author.
E-mail address: abbaseabbas@gmail.com

Surg Clin N Am 101 (2021) 427–441
https://doi.org/10.1016/j.suc.2021.03.005
0039-6109/21/© 2021 Elsevier Inc. All rights reserved.

surgical.theclinics.com

(ACA). For the purposes of this article, EEC is defined as one that is superficial and has no evidence of nodal or distant metastasis (T1-2N0M0).

NATURAL HISTORY OF ESOPHAGEAL CANCER

Although worldwide squamous cell carcinoma is more prevalent, in the United States and most of the Western world ACA is by far the more common form of this disease and has been attributed to gastroesophageal acid reflux disease (GERD) and Barrett esophagus (BE). BE is a metaplastic change of esophageal squamous epithelium into specialized intestinal mucosa in response to acid injury and can advance sequentially from metaplasia to low-grade dysplasia to high-grade dysplasia and then to invasive ACA. Although progression from low-grade dysplasia to high-grade dysplasia may take many years, the average time for high-grade dysplasia to devolve into ACA is only 14 months.[5] Despite this known association of GERD to BE and esophageal cancer, however, up to 45% of BE develops in patients with no symptoms of GERD, and only 10% to 15% of patients diagnosed with esophageal cancer have BE.[6]

DIAGNOSIS AND STAGING OF EARLY ESOPHAGEAL CANCER

Prompt and accurate diagnosis and staging are essential before offering patients appropriate treatments.

Esophagogastroduodenoscopy (EGD) is an endoscopic modality that is particularly useful because it functions as a method of diagnosis, staging, treatment, and surveillance for patients with esophageal cancer. The objective is to determine the location of the tumor with relation of the gastroesophageal junction, tumor length, and degree of luminal obstruction. Additionally, it is important to obtain multiple biopsies (6–8) for sufficient tissue by which to obtain histologic diagnosis and for future molecular analysis (markers, such as PD-L1, HER2neu, and MMR).

Computed tomography (CT) of the chest and abdomen with intravenous and oral contrast remains a cornerstone for esophageal cancer staging. An esophageal wall thickness greater than 5 mm is consistent with T1-2 tumors, 15 mm with T3 tumors, and invasion of adjacent structures with T4 tumors. Unfortunately, the accuracy of CT used for T staging varies widely by study, ranging from 43% to 92%, and CT is unable to distinguish among T1a, T1b, and T2 tumors.[7]

The main role of fluorodeoxyglucose (18F-FDG) PET/CT scanning in initial staging of esophageal cancer lies in its superior ability for detection of distant and regional disease.[8,9] Among primary tumors, 68% to 100% show FDG uptake.[8]

Endoscopic ultrasound (EUS) has become standard of care for staging of esophageal cancer. Compared with various staging modalities, EUS is more accurate in assessing locoregional disease. Sometimes, obstructive bulky tumors do not allow complete assessment by the EUS probe but, in general, EUS is extremely sensitive and specific for accurately predicting T1 versus T3/4 tumors (more than 90% in some studies). In a meta-analysis, Puli and colleagues[10] analyzed the pooled accuracy of EUS in determining the depth of tumor invasion among 42 studies (N = 5039 EUS procedures). Pooled sensitivity rates were 87.8%, 80.5%, 96.4%, and 95.4%, respectively, whereas pooled specificity rates were 98.3%, 95.6%, 90.6%, and 98.3%, respectively, for levels T1, T2, T3, and T4. In the same study, the pooled sensitivity and specificity of EUS for nodal staging were 84.7% and 84.6%, respectively.[10] EUS, however, is reported as less accurate in EEC, reporting a 65% tumor stage concordance between EUS and pathology.[11] It nonetheless is essential to evaluate tumors by EUS prior to any attempted endoscopic resection.

Characterization of nodes by size and appearance (eg echogenicity and irregularity of shape) is key by which to achieve a ultrasonographic TNM stage by the most current American Joint Committee on Cancer classification.

In the authors' practice, for patients planning to undergo a trimodality approach, staging laparoscopy is performed to rule out carcinomatosis and to consider place-ment of a jejunostomy feeding tube. Although placement of a jejunostomy feeding tube may be considered de rigueur after esophagectomy, it also should be considered preoperatively should patients present with severe malnutrition due to dysphagia. Maintaining enteral access may be a key strategy to enable nutrition and hydration for the patient undergoing induction therapy, thus enabling the completion of neoad-juvant therapy without interruption. Nutritional supervision throughout the course of treatment also is critically important to optimize patients preoperatively as well as to counsel them regarding dietary modifications postoperatively.

TREATMENT OF EARLY ESOPHAGEAL CANCER

Most authorities agree that EEC often can be cured with local therapy alone as opposed to intermediate stages, where additional multimodality protocols usually are employed, including surgery, chemotherapy, radiation, and, more recently, immunotherapy.

Endoscopic Therapy for Early Esophageal Cancer

All guidelines, including those of the National Comprehensive Cancer Network (NCCN), recommend that esophagectomy should be considered for all physiologically fit patients with EEC.[12] One caveat is T1a and rare T1b tumors, which are limited to the muscularis mucosa (T1a-MM) or superficial submucosa (T1b-SM1). For those pa-tients, endoscopic mucosal resection, endoscopic submucosal dissection, or endo-scopic ablation, such as with radiofrequency or liquid nitrogen, followed by close surveillance increasingly is offered at experienced centers, with reported oncologic outcomes similar to those of esophagectomy.[13,14]

If the tissue yielded by endoscopic resection shows that resection was incomplete or if the tumor has features that are high-risk factors for invasiveness, however, then surgery should be the recommended treatment. These techniques are discussed in more detail in a separate article.

Inoperable Early Esophageal Cancer

In 2008, Ishikawa and colleagues,[15] published their experience with definitive radiation therapy alone for stage I (Union for International Cancer Control T1N0M0) esophageal squamous cell carcinoma and reported a 5-year disease-free survival rate of 80%. Other modalities that the authors' group and others have employed for inoperable or patients who decline surgery with T1b-T2 tumors include chemoradiation or com-bined endoscopic resectional and ablative therapy (**Fig. 1**).[16]

Esophagectomy

Most approaches to an esophagectomy operation include a transthoracic mediastinal dissection, for example, Ivor Lewis, McKeown, and Sweet, all named after their found-ing surgeons. The transhiatal esophagectomy approach is the only one that does not and relies on transcervical and transabdominal dissection of the intrathoracic esoph-agus. These surgeries commonly are performed "open," that is, through laparotomy and thoracotomy. Over the past 2 decades, however, minimally invasive adaptations of each of these techniques have been described.

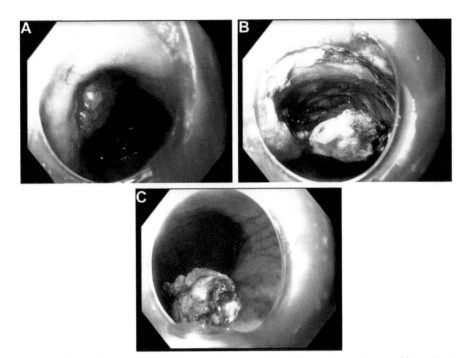

Fig. 1. Endoscopic submucosal dissection for a small T1b tumor in an inoperable patient. Microscopically positive deep margin was managed by additional endoscopic cryospray therapy. (*A*) Endoscopic view of tumor. (*B*) Submucosal dissection, including tumor. (*C*) Resected specimen.

The major benefits of traditional minimally invasive esophagectomy (MIE) by means of standard laparoscopy and thoracoscopy are related to decreased postoperative pain, leading to fewer respiratory complications, faster hospital discharge, and earlier return to normal activities.[17] Several studies have established these and other outcome benefits attributed to MIE, although there still is some controversy regarding the exact degree of advantage.[18–20] There are inherent limitations, however, when sacrificing the open incision approach in favor of traditional keyhole surgery, including rigid instrumentation, the need for a skilled assistant and 2-dimensional imaging, and lack of the ability to perform bimanual dissection. For a complex operation, such as esophagectomy, a surgeon must work with a talented assistant who is able to direct the camera and retract tissues, often from the opposite side of the visual field.

As robotic surgery emerged, its many technical advantages soon were appreciated by surgeons. Having a self-directed stereoscopic camera lying between articulating instruments gives experience similar to open surgery with 3-dimensional vision and bimanual handling, allowing easier complex maneuvers, such as dissection, suturing, and ligation through subcentimeter ports.[21]

The next section discusses the authors' operative approach to the different robotic-assisted MIE (RAMIE) procedures.

OPERATIVE DETAILS FOR ROBOTIC-ASSISTED MINIMALLY INVASIVE ESOPHAGECTOMY
Intraoperative Endoscopic Assessment

Intraoperative endoscopy should be performed for clear anatomic definition of the proximal and distal extent of the tumor and any associated pathology, such as BE.

This has important implications for the surgical approach, location of the anastomosis, and choice of the conduit. For example, a high proximal tumor extension might require a cervical anastomosis for adequate margins. Extension of the tumor onto the cardia or further onto the lesser curvature might render the stomach unusable and require gastrectomy with the use of an alternative conduit.[22]

Bronchoscopy also is performed on the table to clear tracheobronchial secretions and confirm absence of airway invasion by the esophageal tumor, especially for those located in the proximal esophagus or midesophagus.[23]

Anesthesia

Standard administration of general anesthesia is administered. Patients require intra-operative monitoring, including pulse oximetry, arterial line, and urinary catheter. For all procedures except the transhiatal approach, single lung ventilation is required. Although a double-lumen tube is standard in many centers, the authors' preference is for a bronchial blocker because it is less bulky and, therefore, safer while dissecting behind the carina. It also can be removed easily leaving a standard single lumen tube for the abdominal part of the procedure and when short-term postoperative ventilation is required.

Patient Positioning

- Thoracic stage of the operation: the patient is positioned in the left lateral decu-bitus position with slight flexion and 45° anterior tilting in a semiprone position (**Fig. 2**).
- Abdominal stage of the operation: the patient is placed in the supine position and a long, soft, medium-sized gel roll is placed under the left flank and left shoulder. The head is turned to the right, and the skin is prepped from the abdomen to the neck in one field (**Fig. 3**). Before robot docking, the patient is transitioned into steep reverse Trendelenburg position.

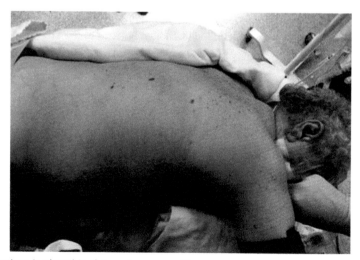

Fig. 2. Patient is placed in the semiprone position.

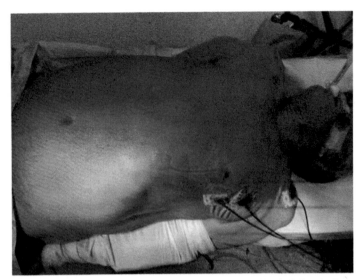

Fig. 3. Patient is placed in the supine position for the cervical and abdominal stages of the operation.

Room Layout

During the procedure, the head of the patient is maintained toward the anesthesia cart and the robot is brought in from the right side of the patient (**Fig. 4**). At the bedside, only a scrub nurse and an assistant are seated, while the operating surgeons are at a dual console.

Port Placement

The authors have standardized thoracic and abdominal port placement for both McKeown and Ivor Lewis procedures.

Thoracic ports
A total of four 8-mm ports and one 12-mm assistant port are placed. The first port is placed at the seventh intercostal space (ICS), just anterior to the anterior axillary line

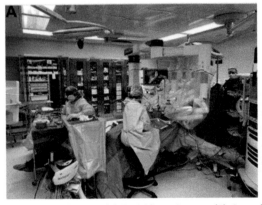
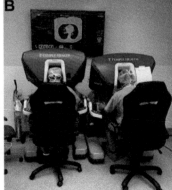

Fig. 4. Room layout. (*A*) Bedside assistants. (*B*) Console surgeons.

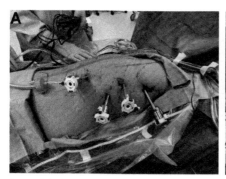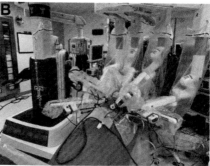

Fig. 5. (A) Thoracic ports are placed as described in the text. (B) Image of thoracic ports after docking.

(Fig. 5). Capnothorax to a pressure of 8 mm Hg to 10 mm Hg is created. A 5-mm thoracoscope is placed and utilized for visual control of the placement of the remaining 3 ports. The camera port is placed at the sixth ICS, with midaxillary line at the midpoint of the thoracic esophagus, approximately 5 cm below the azygos vein arch. Following this, another port is placed in the third ICS, midaxillary line for the right arm, and the final port is placed in the ninth ICS at the posterior axillary line for the left arm. Care should be taken to space the ports appropriately (eg, by 8 cm) to avoid external robotic arm collision. A Vessel Sealer is placed in the right arm, while the left arm will use a bipolar fenestrated grasping forceps. The superior robotic arm is used mainly for retraction, utilizing an atraumatic double fenestrated or tip-up fenestrated forceps. The right hand uses mainly the bipolar Vessel Sealer, alternating with the robotic stapler. The left arm mainly uses the bipolar fenestrated or Cadiere forceps to assist in dissection, exposure, and hemostasis. A 12-mm port is placed in the ninth ICS for assistance.

Abdominal ports
Pneumoperitoneum is created with a Veress needle through the umbilicus. Next, a 12-mm port is placed just below the umbilicus in the midline (**Fig. 6**). The left-hand port is placed at the right midclavicular line, below the costal margin. The camera port is positioned at the left paramedian line, 2 cm below the level of the left-hand port. The 2 remaining ports are placed on the same level. The right-hand port is located in the left midclavicular line and the fourth port for retraction is placed in the left flank. For liver retraction, the authors use a flexible retractor through a 5-mm port in the right flank.

Specific Robotic Esophagectomy Procedures

Modified McKeown esophagectomy
Part 1: right robotic-assisted thoracoscopy. The lung is retracted anteriorly, and the inferior pulmonary ligament is divided (Video 1). The mediastinal pleura is divided longitudinally anterior and posterior to the esophagus up to the level of the azygos vein arch. The vein then is dissected free and usually left intact unless the tumor is bulky. Otherwise, the azygos vein arch is ligated and divided. Both vagus nerves are divided bilaterally as dissection proceeds circumferentially around the upper esophagus to minimize stretch injury to the recurrent laryngeal nerves during the cervical portion of the procedure. The esophagus then is dissected circumferentially, along with all the periesophageal lymph nodes and fatty tissue in between the azygos vein, aorta, and pericardium. Great caution is taken to not incur injury to the thoracic

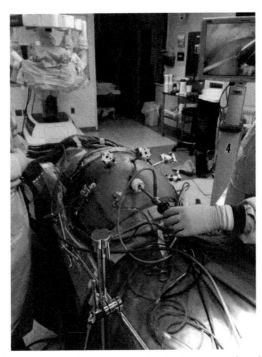

Fig. 6. Robotic-assisted laparoscopic surgery. Abdominal ports are placed as described in the text.

duct. Superior and inferior paratracheal lymph nodes are dissected and removed separately. Penrose drains are encircled around the esophagus at the thoracic inlet and the diaphragm and are tucked under the pleura at either end to be used for retraction during the next stages of the surgery. A flexible 24F drain is placed along the posterior mediastinum. The instruments then are removed, the robot is undocked, and the incisions are closed. The bronchial blocker is removed because the remainder of the procedure does not require lung isolation.

Part 2: left cervicotomy. It is important to complete this part of the procedure before docking the robot and hindering the access to the neck (**Fig. 7**). A 4-cm incision is made along the inferior anterior border of the left sternocleidomastoid muscle. The carotid sheath and internal jugular vein are retracted laterally, and the prevertebral plane is developed. The Penrose drain around the esophagus from thoracic dissection is identified and delivered into the wound.

Part 3: robotic-assisted laparoscopy. During the dissection, the right flank arm is used mainly for retraction utilizing a nontraumatic double fenestrated or tip-up fenestrated grasper (see **Fig. 6**). The right-hand port is used for a majority of the dissection through which the Vessel Sealer also can be used as a needle driver and suture cutter. During pyloromyotomy, this arm is switched for the bipolar Maryland forceps. The left arm uses the fenestrated bipolar or Cadiere forceps to assist in dissection and retraction.

Gastric dissection and conduit preparation are begun by dividing the gastrohepatic ligament and dissection of the diaphragmatic hiatus. The phrenoesophageal ligament is maintained intact until the end of the gastric mobilization in order to minimize loss of

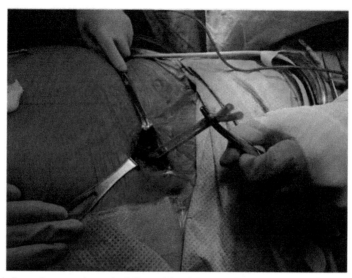

Fig. 7. A left cervicotomy is made followed by delivery of the upper Penrose drain.

pneumoperitoneum into the chest. After identifying the gastroepiploic pedicle, the short gastric vessels and greater omentum are divided in a caudal direction toward the pylorus toward the takeoff of the right gastroepiploic artery from the gastroduodenal artery. Gentle kocherization is completed by dividing lateral retroperitoneal attachments of the duodenum. The authors perform a pyloromyotomy. The stomach then is retracted superiorly, retrogastric adhesions are divided, and left gastric pedicle is identified. After a complete nodal dissection of the nodes around the left gastric, common hepatic, and splenic arteries, the left gastric artery then is divided with the linear stapler at its takeoff from the celiac artery. The lower Penrose drain from the chest then is retrieved and is used for retraction of the gastroesophageal junction. Division of the phrenoesophageal ligament follows, and the authors proceed with formation of the gastric conduit. The nasogastric tube (NGT) is withdrawn into the thoracic esophagus. The stomach is divided with a linear stapler, starting at the incisura and running along the greater curvature to the fundus to form a narrow, 5-cm gastric tube. The perfusion of the gastric conduit can be assessed with indocyanine green (ICG) fluorescence angiography (**Fig. 8**). The fundus is sutured to the distal end of the resected specimen, ready to be delivered into the cervical neck incision. Under visualization by the surgeon at the console, the assistant delivers the esophagogastric specimen along with the attached conduit into the cervicotomy wound. The diaphragmatic hiatus is closed loosely around the conduit with interrupted 3-0 silk suture, and the robot then is undocked. A feeding 12F jejunostomy tube then is advanced through the abdominal wall and passed through a jejunostomy. This then is buried in a subserosal tunnel with interrupted 3-0 suture.

Part 4: delivery of specimen with conduit and cervical anastomosis. The bedside surgeon moves to the neck and pulls on the cervical Penrose drain, which encircles the esophagus to manually deliver the specimen which is attached to the conduit (**Fig. 9**). Once delivered, the conduit length and vascularity are assessed. During this maneuver, the console surgeon watches the conduit carefully to ensure lack of torsion. Once delivered, the hiatus is closed around the conduit in the abdomen. A manual cervical

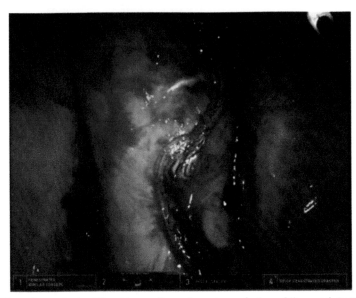

Fig. 8. ICG angiography is utilized to confirm adequate perfusion of the conduit. This image actually shows decreased fluorescence at tip of conduit necessitating adjusting the length of the conduit accordingly.

anastomosis finally is completed, according to surgeon preference. The authors prefer a linear completely stapled side-to-side technique.

Robotic Ivor Lewis esophagectomy
Part 1: robotic-assisted laparoscopy. Gastric dissection and preparation of the gastric conduit are identical to those described previously with the following differences: the conduit remains in the abdomen and the hiatus is not closed (this is performed during the thoracic portion of the procedure) (Video 2).

Part 2: right robotic-assisted thoracoscopy. Until the vagus nerves are divided bilaterally below the recurrent laryngeal nerve takeoff, all the steps are the same as described previously. The specimen and conduit are delivered into the chest. Attention is paid to maintain proper orientation of the conduit to avoid axial torsion during the conduit delivery. The NGT is pulled back to 20 cm, and the esophagus is divided

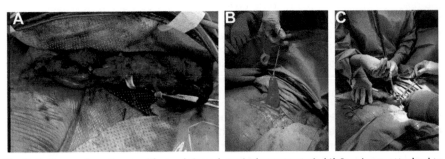

Fig. 9. Delivery of specimen with conduit and cervical anastomosis.(*A*) Specimen attached to the conduit. (*B*) Conduit delivered to the neck with adequate length and vascularity. (*C*) A side-to-side stapled anastomosis is performed with the linear stapler.

with a linear stapler just above the azygos vein arch. The specimen then is delivered from the surgical field through an endobag, and frozen section on the margins is performed to ensure negative margins.

There are different techniques for the formation of the anastomosis. The authors prefer a robotic side-to-side linear stapler technique. Once negative margins are confirmed, the stapled end of the esophagus is opened at the medial end of the staple line. Likewise, a gastrotomy is created in the lateral aspect of the conduit. A 45-mm robotic linear stapler is used. Under direct vision, the NGT is advanced into the caudal portion of the conduit. The esophagogastrostomy edges then are approximated with 2-0 silk stitches before being reinforced by firing another linear stapler.

The diaphragmatic hiatus is closed with interrupted silk stitches around the conduit, which is sutured to the right crus with 2-0 silk. This prevents the future development of paraesophageal hernias.

Finally, a flexible 24F flexible drain is placed along the posterior esophageal gutter. The robotic instruments then are removed, the robot is undocked, and the incisions are closed.

Robotic transhiatal esophagectomy

The robotic transhiatal esophagectomy technique has been described by other investigators.[24]

Part 1: abdominal part of the procedure. The gastric dissection and preparation of the gastric conduit are identical to those described previously, with the following differences.

The circumferential dissection of the esophagus proceeds proximally with care to include all periesophageal tissue. In cases of the pleural cavities entered, the pleura is immediately repaired with either a clip or a running simple suture in order to minimize loss of pneumoperitoneum. The dissection is carried as proximally as possible along the esophagus, taking full advantage of the multi-articulating instruments, tremor reduction, and 2-dimensional visualization that the robotic platform offers.

Part 2: left cervicotomy. Left cervicotomy can be done simultaneously with the abdominal part. Careful exposure and circumferential dissection of the cervical esophagus are performed in caudal direction until the esophagus is completely freed from below and above. Care must be taken to avoid injury of the recurrent laryngeal nerves because the vagus nerves have not been separated from the esophagus as is done in the McKeown procedure. Often, the bedside surgeon can see and feel the robotic instrument in the mediastinum. After delivery of the conduit, the procedure proceeds in similar steps to the left cervicotomy, described previously.

POSTOPERATIVE MANAGEMENT

Patients are extubated in the immediate postoperative period and typically remain in the hospital until their thoracic and nasogastric drains are removed. This usually is achieved by postoperative days 5 to 7. They are discharged home on enteral nutrition via the jejunal tube. A water-soluble esophagram is performed as an outpatient procedure approximately 2 weeks after surgery. When an esophageal leak is ruled out, the patient is advanced to an oral diet. The diet is advanced progressively until full caloric intake is met via oral route. At this point, enteral nutrition is ceased.[23] Postoperatively, patients are advised of lifestyle and diet modifications, such as scheduling small frequent meals, avoiding eating before bedtime, sleeping with the head of bed elevated, and possibly using proton pump inhibitors.[25]

FOLLOW-UP

Per NCCN guidelines, differences in follow-up for early-stage esophageal cancer reflect a spectrum of heterogeneous potential for locoregional relapse and overall survival (OS). Most recurrences occur within 24 months of initial treatment. Regarding early-stage esophageal cancer, recommendations for surveillance vary according to the depth of invasion and treatment modality used. There are stage-specific guidelines for surveillance based on recommended imaging and intervals of follow-up, but the surveillance strategies remain controversial without high-level evidence for guidance.

In general, patients who undergo endoscopic resection of EEC (cTis-T1a) should undergo EGD every 3 months for the first year, every 6 months for the second year, and annually thereafter. There is no strict recommendation for CT imaging in this patient population. Patients who undergo more definitive surgical treatment are subject to less frequent CT chest/abdomen imaging guidelines. For example, patients who undergo esophagectomy for early-stage esophageal cancer (cT1b, any N) are advised to undergo CT chest/abdomen with intravenous contrast every 12 months for up to 3 years; there are no specific recommendations to perform EGD in these patients.[26] For those who undergo esophagectomy in the setting of multimodal treatment (cT2-T4, any N), CT surveillance imaging is recommended every 6 months for 2 years, with EGD on an as-needed basis.

OUTCOMES

Despite the established superiority of esophagectomy over other modalities in terms of oncologic outcomes, it is a major operation, which is designed for removing and replacing an organ that traverses 3 body cavities, hence the difficulty and potential for morbidity. These risks have decreased over time thanks to improvement in surgical techniques and hospital care. Postoperative complications after esophagectomy consistently have been shown to be less frequent and more successfully managed in higher-volume hospitals.[27] Postoperative complications after esophagectomy are influenced by many factors, including patient comorbidities, other treatments, the operative approach, and the learning curve. Both MIE and RAMIE share the same potential risks of open esophagectomy, including the potential for infection, bleeding, and cardiopulmonary complications. Moreover, there are additional risks that are unique to the robotic platform.[28]

The authors published experience of 33 robotic esophagectomies in 2013.[22] Postoperative complications developed in 39% of patients, with anastomotic leaks and chylothorax in 6% each. Mortality occurred in 1 (3%) patient on postoperative day 12 due to mesenteric ischemia. Since that time, the RAMIE experience has expanded to become a predominant approach for esophagectomy at major centers. Kingma and colleagues,[29] in their review, found that RAMIE, when compared with open esophagectomy, was associated with less intraoperative blood loss, lower postoperative pain scores, faster functional recovery, and better quality of life. There were no significant differences regarding lymph node yield and OS between the open, MIE, and RAMIE groups, which suggests that RAMIE maintains equal oncologic efficacy to the other approaches for esophagectomy.[29] Other investigators have compared MIE versus RAMIE and found that both had similar results in terms of adequacy of cancer resection, comparing negative margins and median lymph node examined, having 98% versus 96% of negative resection margins and 19 versus 26 median lymph nodes examined, respectively. Anastomotic leak was 5% versus 4% for MIE and RAMIE, respectively. Ultimately, 30-day mortality was 1.7% in the MIE group versus 0% in the RAMIE group.[30]

In 2017, Park and colleagues,[31] in a follow-up analysis, reported on the oncologic feasibility of the robotic-assisted technique. OS at 3 years was 85% and recurrence-free survival was 79.4%. Subgroup analysis demonstrated 3-year OS was 94.4% in patients with stage I disease, 86.2% in patients with stage II disease, 77.8% in patients with stage IIIA disease, and 37.5% in patients with stage IIIB disease. The 3-year recurrence-free survival was 96.2% in patients with stage I disease, 80.1% in patients with stage II disease, and 79.5% in patients with stage IIIA disease. Such examples of excellent outcomes rival and possibly exceed those achieved by more traditional approaches in preceding eras.[31]

CLINICS CARE POINTS

The following are useful surgical pearls during an esophagectomy:

- Use of ICG and robotic fluorescence imaging is helpful to guide the assessment of viability in the creation of the gastric conduit

- Considerations to use possible omental flap as a buttress can be applied to the intrathoracic anastomosis during the Ivor Lewis approach.

- Great caution should be taken to avoid direct or delayed injury to the left mainstem bronchus and carina with use of energy devices during subcarinal nodal dissection. A bronchial blocker may be less bulky and safer in this regard.

- It is important to purposely divide both vagal nerves along the proximal esophagus while dissecting along the proximal esophagus while dissecting this area so that inadvertent traction on the recurrent laryngeal nerves (during left cervical neck dissection) is avoided.

- The posterior mediastinal drain around the intrathoracic anastomosis during the Ivor Lewis approach should be positioned carefully so as to not lie immediately adjacent to the anastomosis, because continuous suction may contribute to the development of an anastomotic leak, albeit contained.

- Postoperative development of paraconduit hernia may be prevented by judicious placement of sutures to close the hiatus after the completion of esophagogastric anastomosis and the gastric conduit has been placed in its final configuration.

- Postoperative esophagrams should explicitly address both the presence of an anastomotic leak and the adequacy of gastric emptying.

- There is no high-level evidence to support the optimal approach to address possible delayed gastric emptying. As such, performing pyloromyotomy (as is the authors' preference), pyloroplasty, or no drainage procedure may be chosen. Alternatively, injection of botulinum toxin (endoscopic or laparoscopic), 100 U, is a simple procedure that carries minimal risk.

SUMMARY

Esophageal cancer is the eighth most common cancer worldwide, and its incidence has been increasing over the past several decades. Endoscopic treatments have demonstrated safety and effectiveness in achieving curative rates only for preinvasive and superficial esophageal cancer. Esophagectomy currently is the standard of care for more advanced EEC and should be performed at centers of excellence with high volumes, appropriate supportive staff, and multidisciplinary expertise. RAMIE has demonstrated efficacy and safety as a minimally invasive approach in comparison with other approaches and when indicated is a valid option for the treatment of EEC. Differences in follow-up for early-stage esophageal cancer reflect a heterogeneous potential for relapse and OS. Consequently, follow-up recommendations vary according to the depth of invasion and treatment modality.

DISCLOSURE

The authors have no potential conflicts of interest.

SUPPLEMENTARY DATA

Supplementary data related to this article can be found online at https://doi.org/10.1016/j.suc.2021.03.005.

REFERENCES

1. Kamangar F, Dores GM, Anderson WF. Patterns of cancer incidence, mortality, and prevalence across five continents: defining priorities to reduce cancer disparities in different geographic regions of the world. J Clin Oncol 2006;24(14):2137–50.
2. Antoni S, Soerjomataram I, Møller B, et al. An assessment of GLOBOCAN methods for deriving national estimates of cancer incidence. Bull World Health Organ 2016;94(3):174–84.
3. SEER Cancer Statistics Review (CSR) 1975-2014. April 2, 2018.
4. Fabian T, Federico JA. The impact of minimally invasive esophageal surgery. Surg Clin North Am 2017;97(4):763–70.
5. Reid BJ, Blount L, Rubin E, et al. Flow-cytometric and histological progression to malignancy in Barrett's esophagus: prospective endoscopic surveillance of a cohort. 8.
6. Zakko L, Lutzke L, Wang KK. Screening and Preventive Strategies in Esophagogastric Cancer. Surg Oncol Clin N Am 2017;26(2):163–78.
7. Bunting D, Bracey T, Fox B, et al. Loco-regional staging accuracy in oesophageal cancer—How good are we in the modern era? Eur J Radiol 2017;97:71–5.
8. Goel R, Subramaniam RM, Wachsmann JW. PET/Computed Tomography scanning and precision medicine. PET Clin 2017;12(4):373–91.
9. Varghese TK, Hofstetter WL, Rizk NP, et al. The society of thoracic surgeons guidelines on the diagnosis and staging of patients with esophageal cancer. Ann Thorac Surg 2013;96(1):346–56.
10. Puli SR, Reddy JB, Bechtold ML, et al. Staging accuracy of esophageal cancer by endoscopic ultrasound: a meta-analysis and systematic review. World J Gastroenterol 2008;14(10):1479.
11. Young PE, Gentry AB, Acosta RD, et al. Endoscopic ultrasound does not accurately stage early adenocarcinoma or high-grade dysplasia of the esophagus. Clin Gastroenterol Hepatol 2010;8(12):1037–41.
12. Ajani JA, Barthel JS, Bentrem DJ, et al. Esophageal and Esophagogastric Junction Cancers. J Natl Compr Canc Netw 2011;9(8):830–87.
13. Larghi A, Lightdale CJ, Memeo L, et al. EUS followed by EMR for staging of high-grade dysplasia and early cancer in Barrett's esophagus. 8.
14. Naveed M, Kubiliun N. Endoscopic treatment of early-stage esophageal cancer. Curr Oncol Rep 2018;20(9):71.
15. Ishikawa H, Sakurai H, Tamaki Y, et al. Radiation therapy alone for stage I (UICC T1N0M0) squamous cell carcinoma of the esophagus: Indications for surgery or combined chemoradiotherapy. J Gastroenterol Hepatol 2006;21(8):1290–6.

16. Tsai FC, Ghorbani S, Greenwald BD, et al. Safety and efficacy of endoscopic spray cryotherapy for esophageal cancer. Dis Esophagus 2017;30(11):1–7.
17. Abbas A, Dylewski MR. Robotic assisted minimally invasive esophagectomy. In: Kim KC, editor. Robotics in general surgery. Springer Science & Business Media; 2013.
18. Luketich JD, Pennathur A, Awais O, et al. Outcomes after minimally invasive esophagectomy: review of over 1000 patients. Ann Surg 2012;256(1):95–103.
19. Biere SSAY, van Berge Henegouwen MI, Maas KW, et al. Minimally invasive versus open oesophagectomy for patients with oesophageal cancer: a multicentre, open-label, randomised controlled trial. Lancet 2012;379(9829):1887–92.
20. Yibulayin W, Abulizi S, Lv H, et al. Minimally invasive oesophagectomy versus open esophagectomy for resectable esophageal cancer: a meta-analysis. World J Surg Oncol 2016;14(1):304.
21. Mazzei M, Abbas AE. Why comprehensive adoption of robotic assisted thoracic surgery is ideal for both simple and complex lung resections. J Thorac Dis 2020; 12(2):70–81.
22. Abbas AE, Dylewski MR. Robotic assisted minimally invasive esophagectomy. In: Kim KC, editor. Robotics in general surgery. New York, NY: Springer New York; 2014. p. 25–32.
23. Petrov RV, Bakhos CT, Abbas AE. Robotic Esophagectomy. In: Tsuda S, Kudsi OY, editors. Robotic-assisted minimally invasive surgery. New York, NY: Springer International Publishing; 2019. p. 277–93.
24. DeLong JC, Kelly KJ, Jacobsen GR, et al. The benefits and limitations of robotic assisted transhiatal esophagectomy for esophageal cancer. J Vis Surg 2016; 2:156.
25. Schmidt HM, Gisbertz SS, Moons J, et al. Defining benchmarks for transthoracic esophagectomy: a multicenter analysis of total minimally invasive esophagectomy in low risk patients. Ann Surg 2017;266(5):814–21.
26. Shaheen NJ, Falk GW, Iyer PG, et al. ACG clinical guideline: diagnosis and management of Barrett's esophagus. Am J Gastroenterol 2016;111(1):30–50.
27. Markar SR, Karthikesalingam A, Thrumurthy S, et al. Volume-outcome relationship in surgery for esophageal malignancy: systematic review and meta-analysis 2000-2011. J Gastrointest Surg 2012;16(5):1055–63.
28. Abbas AE, Sarkaria IS. Specific complications and limitations of robotic esophagectomy. Dis Esophagus 2020;33(Supplement_2).
29. Kingma BF, de Maat MFG, van der Horst S, et al. Robot-assisted minimally invasive esophagectomy (RAMIE) improves perioperative outcomes: a review. J Thorac Dis 2019;11(S5):S735–42.
30. Okusanya OT, Sarkaria IS, Hess NR, et al. Robotic assisted minimally invasive esophagectomy (RAMIE): the University of Pittsburgh Medical Center initial experience. Ann Cardiothorac Surg 2017;6(2):179–85.
31. Park SY, Kim DJ, Do YW, et al. The oncologic outcome of esophageal squamous cell carcinoma patients after robot-assisted thoracoscopic esophagectomy with total mediastinal lymphadenectomy. Ann Thorac Surg 2017;103(4):1151–7.

Chemoradiation Therapy as Definitive Treatment of Esophageal Cancer

Sue Xue Wang, MD[a], M. Blair Marshall, MD[a,b,*]

KEYWORDS

- Esophageal carcinoma • Definitive chemoradiation • Multimodality therapy
- Immunotherapy

KEY POINTS

- There are significant differences in tumor treatment response and recurrence patterns in esophageal squamous cell cancer compared with adenocarcinoma.
- The role of surgery after chemoradiation is debated in patients with squamous cell cancer, whereas multimodality therapy including surgery is currently the standard in adenocarcinoma.
- Better understanding of cancer biology and targeted therapy is evolving the treatment of esophageal cancer.

INTRODUCTION

Trimodality therapy is the current standard of care for the management of patients with advanced esophageal cancer. However, this standard may be in the process of evolution. Given the success of definitive chemoradiation therapy (dCRT) in cervical esophageal cancer as well as concern for the perioperative and long-term morbidity of esophagectomy,[1] the role of dCRT in thoracic esophageal cancer has been increasingly contemplated. In addition, the increased use of PET in defining response to treatment as well as the consideration of variances in response of specific esophageal cancer histology has allowed the oncologic management of this pathology to become more nuanced. Some studies have shown dCRT to result in a complete pathologic response in 20% to 25% of patients or to have matched long-term survival compared with treatment combinations where surgery plays a critical role.[2,3] In patients who are medically unfit for esophagectomy, dCRT is the treatment of choice. For cervical esophageal

[a] Division of Thoracic Surgery, Brigham and Women's Hospital, 75 Francis Street, Boston, MA 02115, USA; [b] Division of Thoracic Surgery, West Roxbury VA Medical Center, 1400 VFW Pkwy, West Roxbury, MA 02132, USA
* Corresponding author. Division of Thoracic Surgery, Brigham and Women's Hospital, 75 Francis Street, Boston, MA 02115.
E-mail address: mmarshall16@bwh.harvard.edu

Surg Clin N Am 101 (2021) 443–451
https://doi.org/10.1016/j.suc.2021.03.006
0039-6109/21/© 2021 Elsevier Inc. All rights reserved.

cancer, extending from the hypopharynx to the sternal notch, dCRT is the standard of care.[4] It is also used in the management of advanced locoregional disease, including potentially resectable (T4a) and unresectable (T4b) primary disease.[5] As multimodality therapy for esophageal cancer continues to evolve, this article presents the current data in support of and against dCRT as primary treatment of esophageal cancer.

ARGUMENT FOR DEFINITIVE CHEMORADIATION THERAPY

Several randomized controlled trials have attempted to hone in on the optimal chemoradiation regimen for patients undergoing dCRT. RTOG 85-01 is a multiinstitutional randomized controlled trial that established that combined chemoradiation therapy significantly increased overall survival compared with radiotherapy alone, with radiation dose escalation providing no additional benefit. Although the study included both esophageal squamous cell carcinoma (SCC) and adenocarcinoma, stage T1-3 N0-1 M0, it is notable that greater than 80% of the research population had squamous cell histology. The 2 arms of the study were (1) definitive chemoradiation using 5-fluorouracil (5-FU) plus cisplatin with 50 Gy and (2) radiation alone using 64 Gy. The chemoradiation arm showed a clear survival benefit resulting in early termination of the study. Five-year overall survival was a respectable 26% (95% confidence interval [CI], 15%–37%) for the chemoradiation arm compared with 0% for the radiation arm.[6] Several additional randomized trials examined alternate radiation or chemotherapy modalities. In patients with clinical stage T1-4 N0-1 M0 esophageal squamous cell (85%) or adenocarcinoma (15%), INT 0123 compared chemoradiation (5-FU and cisplatin) in combination with either the standard 50.4 Gy radiation therapy or higher 64.8 Gy radiation therapy. The researchers found no difference in survival or locoregional control. This study established 50.4 Gy as the definitive radiation therapy dose for patients treated with concurrent 5-FU and cisplatin chemotherapy.[7] The PRODIGE5/ACCORD17 trial substituted the FOLFOX regimen (5-FU, oxaliplatin, leucovorin) for 5-FU and cisplatin with similar survival rates and reduced chemotherapy toxicity.[8]

Two randomized control trials compared chemoradiotherapy with and without surgery and found no significant difference in overall survival. Stahl and colleagues conducted a phase III study including 172 patients with locally advanced esophageal SCC. The surgery arm demonstrated much higher treatment-related mortality (30-day mortality 12.8%, in-hospital mortality 11.3%) compared with the dCRT arm (30-day mortality 3.5%, $P = .03$). Overall survival at 2 years was equivalent between the surgery (39.9% CI, 29.4%–50.4%) and dCRT (35.4 %CI, 25.2%–45.6%) arms. However, it should be noted that disease-free survival was superior in the surgery arm with 2-year disease-free survival of 64.3% (95% CI, 52.1%–76.5%) compared with 40.7% (95% CI, 28.9%–52.5%) in the dCRT arm.[2] Another study by Bedenne and colleagues included 259 patients with operable T3 N0-1 M0 thoracic esophageal cancer with 88% SCC histology. The 3-month mortality rate was again higher in the surgery arm at 9.3% compared with 0.8% in the dCRT arm.[3] As a result of these studies, chemoradiation followed by surgery compared with chemoradiation alone are considered equivalent for survival in locally advanced esophageal SCC.

If there is no significant survival difference between patients treated with dCRT compared with trimodality therapy, it is desirable to avoid the short- and long-term morbidity of esophagectomy. Definitive chemoradiation is the treatment of choice for patients who are medically unfit for esophagectomy. Patients may be considered medically unfit due to overall frailty, poor pulmonary reserve, or cardiac comorbidities. The perioperative complications of esophagectomy are substantial, including anastomotic leak, recurrent laryngeal nerve injury, pneumonia, and myocardial infarction.[9]

Postoperatively, many patients continue to have functional gastrointestinal disorders including dysphagia from strictures, delayed gastric emptying, reflux, and postgastrectomy dumping syndrome.[10] We acknowledge that medically frail patients also have difficulty tolerating chemoradiation, with a retrospective study in elderly patients with esophageal cancer (age >75 years, n = 89) showing that 20% required radiation therapy breaks, 37% had a chemotherapy dose reduction, and 39.5% had a cycle reduction. Of this group, 15% were unable to complete radiation therapy and 22% experienced acute grade 3+ toxicity.[11]

Furthermore, current advances in radiation techniques suggest a trend toward improved treatment outcomes. Yamaguchi and colleagues investigated induction chemotherapy followed by either dCRT or surgery for T4 esophageal cancer with tracheobronchial invasion. It remains controversial and institution dependent whether surgical resection or definitive chemoradiation should be performed after induction chemotherapy. No significant difference in survival was observed between the 2 arms, but the study demonstrated improved prognosis in patients receiving dCRT from 2006 to 2013 compared with those receiving dCRT from 2003 to 2006. During the later treatment period, the institution adopted new 3-dimensional (3D) radiation planning techniques.[12] Additional advances in radiation dosing, including intensity-modulated radiation therapy[13] or 4D computed tomography (CT) could further improve dCRT outcomes by increasing selectivity in radiation dose delivery.

After treatment with chemoradiation, some patients are noted to have a pathologic complete response; these patients may not require surgery to be cured of their disease. In the CROSS trial, 49% of patients with SCC and 23% with adenocarcinoma achieved pathologic complete response.[14] Clinical complete response after neoadjuvant chemoradiotherapy has been correlated with pathologic complete response in 72.7% of patients. This population had significantly better 3-year overall survival than nonclinical complete responders.[15] Clinical complete responses are noted to be more common in SCC, women, and tumors with lower T stages and poor differentiation.[16] Currently, an active surveillance protocol is being studied where patients with complete clinical response undergo routine surveillance after completion of chemoradiotherapy and receive surgery only if needed.[17]

Should patients undergo dCRT and develop local recurrence, several studies suggest salvage esophagectomy is a feasible treatment strategy for medically fit patients. RTOG-0246 was a nonrandomized phase II study of patients with T1-4N0M0 esophageal adenocarcinoma or SCC. Patients received induction chemotherapy for 2 cycles (5-FU, cisplatin, paclitaxel) followed by dCRT (5-FU with 50.4 Gy). Patients were offered salvage esophagectomy for residual or recurrent disease after dCRT with a 5-year survival rate of 36.6% (95% CI, 22.3–51.0). In a separate multicenter retrospective study, neoadjuvant chemotherapy followed by surgery versus definitive chemoradiation followed by salvage esophagectomy were found to have no difference in disease-free survival or overall survival. Although there was no survival difference, the salvage esophagectomy group had a significantly higher incidence of postoperative anastomotic leak (17.2% vs 10.7%) and surgical site infection. Salvage esophagectomy for persistent disease had a lower overall survival than salvage esophagectomy for recurrent disease, again suggesting that responders and nonresponders to dCRT have different patterns of disease.[18]

ARGUMENT AGAINST DEFINITIVE CHEMORADIATION THERAPY

Our current understanding of the treatment of esophageal cancer is derived from research with considerable limitations. Many of the pioneering trials in this field are only just adequately powered, containing only 100 or 200 patients. Esophageal cancer is a rare disease, and in order to enroll enough patients, many of the studies reviewed grouped together squamous and adenocarcinoma histologies, not accounting for their biological differences in patterns of recurrence, response to treatment, and survival outcomes. Evidence dividing esophageal adenocarcinoma and squamous cell cancer continues to grow. The research discussed to date emphasized primarily squamous cell disease. Furthermore, because of their age, much of the existing research guiding treatment in esophageal cancer did not incorporate PET as part of their oncologic evaluation, limiting their ability to detect distant metastases. As a result of the understandable limitations in power and study design, similar trials in this field report contradictory outcomes, contributing to controversy in esophageal cancer treatment.

Although the role of surgery after chemoradiation is debated in patients with squamous cell cancer, surgical resection is generally recommended for patients with adenocarcinoma. Adenocarcinoma is less sensitive to chemoradiation than squamous cell cancer. Again, in the CROSS trial, 23% (28/121) of patients with adenocarcinoma compared with 49% (18/37, $P = .008$) of patients with SCC were observed to have a pathologic complete response.[14] Even in squamous cell histology, disease-free survival was superior after surgery due to high rates of local recurrence following chemoradiation with curative intent.[2] Multiple studies found that the prevalence of distant metastasis following dCRT is significantly higher in adenocarcinoma than in SCC,[19,20] as high as 48% in adenocarcinoma compared with 27.5% in SCC.[20] Local recurrence after dCRT in SCC could feasibly be treated with observation and salvage esophagectomy. However, the increased risk of distant metastasis in adenocarcinoma would limit the patient to palliative therapy with dismal outcomes.

Adenocarcinoma is less likely to show complete pathologic response than esophageal SCC. Predictors of disease recurrence after complete pathologic response were:

- Adenocarcinoma histology
- Tumors T3 or greater
- Poorly differentiated tumors
- Positive lymph nodes
- Retreatment standard uptake value (SUV) greater than 10[20]

An estimated 20% to 40% of patients with complete response will have a recurrence within 2 years.[20] Amini and colleagues retrospectively identified 141 patients who obtained initial clinical complete response after dCRT for esophageal cancer. Of this group, 55% of patients experienced disease recurrence at median follow-up of 22 months (range 6–87 months).[21] Moreover, it is not possible to reliably identify patients with complete pathologic response by PET or endoscopy. A retrospective study by Port and colleagues observed that the false-negative rate of PET postinduction is higher than before therapy and should be interpreted with caution. They found that 66% of patients with an SUV of 2.5 or less still had viable tumor on surgical resection, and 64% of patients with node-negative scans were found to have positive lymph nodes.[22] Esophageal ultrasound is also less accurate for restaging after radiation and chemotherapy, as it is difficult to distinguish inflammation and fibrosis from residual cancer on biopsy.[23] Posttreatment staging and monitoring of complete clinic response carries significant limitations, highlighting the importance of pretreatment patient selection and understanding factors that predict failure of the various treatment modalities.

Just as there have been advances in radiation techniques, advances in surgical technique with increased case volume of esophagectomy, experience with perioperative management, and a transition toward minimally invasive techniques have decreased the morbidity of esophagectomy. In comparison to Stahl and colleagues's[2] in-hospital mortality rate of 11.3% seen during 1994 to 2002, perioperative mortality was only 3.4% following esophagectomy in the Society of Thoracic Surgeon's analysis on cases from 2011 to 2014.[24] This discrepancy limits generalizability to the present day and suggests possible survival benefit in high-volume esophagectomy centers with low mortality. Furthermore, 34% of the induction-followed-by-surgery arm in Stahl's paper did not proceed with surgery and there was incomplete tumor resection in 18% of total patients. They also noted superior disease-free survival in the surgery arm despite equivalent overall survival. The association between surgery and survival benefit persists even with locally advanced adenocarcinoma. Raman and colleagues used the National Cancer Database to identify 182 patients with clinical T4a N0-3 M0 esophageal adenocarcinoma who were treated between 2010 and 2015. Propensity matching was performed for 63 patient pairs who underwent surgery following perioperative chemotherapy compared with dCRT and demonstrated a significant survival benefit (hazard ratio 0.26; 95% CI 0.16–0.43).[25] With recent dramatic improvements in perioperative mortality in esophagectomy, coupled with superior disease-free survival in the treatment arms including surgery, we could argue that surgery plays an irreplaceable role in the treatment of esophageal cancer.

More recent studies are less likely to equate dCRT and trimodality therapy. The landmark CROSS trial in 2012 established the role of neoadjuvant chemoradiotherapy followed by surgery for resectable locally advanced disease as standard of care. The analysis included 75% adenocarcinoma histology.[14] In 2017, Van Ruler and colleagues conducted a retrospective, 2-center study in the Netherlands evaluating outcomes following definitive chemoradiation in 66 patients who were poor surgical candidates and had resectable, locally advanced disease. Treatment consisted of carboplatin and paclitaxel with 50.4 Gy. However, median survival was only 13.1 months with a 2-year overall survival of 30%. At 2 years, 26% (95% CI 15%–37%) of patients had developed local progression and 49% (95% CI 36%–64%) had distant metastases. These outcomes are inferior to reported outcomes of trimodality therapy.[26] Despite the limited size of this study, it suggests that every effort should be made to optimize marginal patients with resectable disease for surgery.

FUTURE CONSIDERATIONS

Cancer treatment is becoming increasingly targeted toward individual tumor biology and patient genetics. The Cancer Genome Atlas analysis demonstrated that adenocarcinomas of the distal esophagus, gastroesophageal junction, and proximal stomach are molecularly closely related[27] and distinct from esophageal SCC. As we enter the era of personalized medicine, molecular and gene profiling will be the guide to defining subsets of patients who should receive specific therapies. Several recent studies are investigating immunotherapy alone versus combination chemotherapy with the addition of a biological agent in the treatment of gastric and distal esophageal adenocarcinoma.

The Trastuzumab for Gastric Cancer (ToGA) trial was an international, phase III, randomized controlled trial that examined trastuzumab in combination with chemotherapy compared with chemotherapy alone in patients with HER2 positive gastroesophageal and esophageal cancer. Trastuzumab combination therapy demonstrated significantly increased overall survival with 13.8 months (95% CI 12–

16) compared with 11.1 months (95% CI 10–13) in the chemotherapy alone arm.[28] The KEYNOTE-059 trial enrolled 259 patients and showed a median response duration of 16.3 months in patients with programmed cell death ligand-1 (PD-L1) positive adeno-carcinoma compared with 6.9 months in patients with PD-L1 negative tumors.[29] The S0356 trial analyzed messenger RNA from esophageal adenocarcinoma treated with oxaliplatin, FU, and concurrent radiotherapy,[30] identifying that expression of the repair gene ERCCI is associated with worse progression-free and overall survival. In our understanding of biological heterogeneity, they are progressing from separating histologies of esophageal cancer into the early days of gene analysis within known histologic subtypes.

SUMMARY

The treatment of esophageal cancer continues to evolve, with immunotherapy, chemoradiation, and surgery all serving essential roles. An individualized and multidisciplinary approach is necessary to provide patients with favorable long-term outcomes. Much of our present knowledge is based on poor-quality studies that mixed esophageal SCC and adenocarcinoma histologies to achieve sufficient power. In current practice, definitive chemoradiation is considered appropriate treatment of patients with locoregionally advanced esophageal SCC, whereas multimodal therapy including surgery is preferred for esophageal adenocarcinoma. However, we are only now beginning to understand the implications of targeted therapy and molecular biology in cancer treatment. More specifically, the role of these therapies in the management of esophageal cancer is in its infancy. We have more questions than answers at this point, and our understanding of esophageal cancer treatment will continue to evolve. As the pendulum swings toward precision medicine through molecular profiling and minimally invasive interventions, we will likely progress to an increased esophageal-sparing approach in a subset of patients whose survival is not improved by the addition of an esophagectomy.

PERSONAL PERSPECTIVE (SENIOR AUTHOR)

Decision-making is the critical component that cannot be gleaned from the available data concerning multimodal management of patients with esophageal cancer. If the literature is flawed on many levels, what are we left with? My personal approach is a watch and wait approach to the management of squamous cell cancers of the esophagus. Because of the changes in radiation modeling as well as the effectiveness of combined chemo/radiation therapy in treating cervical squamous cell cancers of the esophagus, we now observe many of these patients. This is if they seem to have a complete response based on PET and endoscopy, which is further supported by a concurrent improvement in surgical techniques with a decrease in morbidity and mortality associated with esophagectomy, even salvage esophagectomy. However, this contrasts with our approach for adenocarcinoma of the esophagus; until there are more data on radically different therapeutic agents, minimally invasive/robotic esophagectomy following neoadjuvant therapy is our standard. Even with a complete response on PET, it has been my observation that often, persistent malignant disease is found in the surgical pathology or recurrence is common in those who wait. Recommendations to follow patients rather than proceed with surgical resection is unsupported. As an exception, it may at times be reasonable to be conservative and follow elderly or frail patients who are at higher risk for an operation.

CLINICS CARE POINTS FOR DEFINITIVE CHEMORADIATION

- Definitive chemoradiation is the standard of care in cervical esophageal cancer, extending from the hypopharynx to the sternal notch.
- The standard definitive chemoradiation regimen is cisplatin/5-FU and 50.4 Gy.
- Patients who are medically unfit for esophagectomy due to frailty, poor pulmonary reserve, or cardiac comorbidities receive definitive chemoradiation.
- Radiation should be administered using selective dose delivery methods such as 3D conformational techniques or intensity-modulated radiation therapy with mapping through 4D CT.
- There are significant differences in tumor treatment response and recurrence patterns in esophageal squamous cell cancer compared with adenocarcinoma that are not completely understood.
- Adenocarcinoma is less sensitive to chemoradiation than squamous cell cancer with higher rates of distant metastasis.
- The role of surgery after chemoradiation is debated in patients with squamous cell cancer, whereas multimodality therapy including surgery is currently the standard in adenocarcinoma.
- Patients with SCC and pathologic complete response could be considered for definitive chemoradiotherapy with close surveillance, although posttreatment with PET and endoscopy is imperfect. Long-term trial data on this approach are still pending.
- Salvage esophagectomy for residual or recurrent disease after definitive chemoradiation should be considered and has been demonstrated to have no difference in disease-free survival or overall survival compared with trimodality therapy.
- Better understanding of cancer biology and targeted therapy is evolving the treatment of esophageal cancer.

DISCLOSURE

The authors have nothing to disclose.

REFERENCES

1. Rutegård M, Lagergren P, Rouvelas I, et al. Surgical complications and long-term survival after esophagectomy for cancer in a nationwide Swedish cohort study. Eur J Surg Oncol 2012;38(7):555–61.
2. Stahl M, Stuschke M, Lehmann N, et al. Chemoradiation with and without surgery in patients with locally advanced squamous cell carcinoma of the esophagus. J Clin Oncol 2005;23(10):2310–7.
3. Bedenne L, Michel P, Bouché O, et al. Chemoradiation followed by surgery compared with chemoradiation alone in squamous cancer of the esophagus: FFCD 9102. J Clin Oncol 2007;25(10):1160–8.
4. Hoeben A, Polak J, Van De Voorde L, et al. Cervical esophageal cancer: a gap in cancer knowledge. Ann Oncol 2016;27(9):1664–74.
5. Jeene PM, van Laarhoven HWM, Hulshof MCCM. The role of definitive chemoradiation in patients with non-metastatic oesophageal cancer. Best Pract Res Clin Gastroenterol 2018;36-37:53–9.

6. Cooper JS, Guo MD, Herskovic A, et al. Chemoradiotherapy of locally advanced esophageal cancer: long-term follow-up of a prospective randomized trial (RTOG 85-01). JAMA 1999;281(17). https://doi.org/10.1001/jama.281.17.1623.

7. Minsky BD, Pajak TF, Ginsberg RJ, et al. INT 0123 (radiation therapy oncology group 94-05) phase III trial of combined-modality therapy for esophageal cancer: high-dose versus standard-dose radiation therapy. J Clin Oncol 2002;20(5): 1167–74.

8. Conroy T, Galais M-P, Raoul J-L, et al. Definitive chemoradiotherapy with FOLFOX versus fluorouracil and cisplatin in patients with oesophageal cancer (PRO-DIGE5/ACCORD17): final results of a randomised, phase 2/3 trial. Lancet Oncol 2014;15(3):305–14.

9. Seely AJE, Ivanovic J, Threader J, et al. Systematic classification of morbidity and mortality after thoracic surgery. Ann Thorac Surg 2010;90(3):936–42.

10. Bailey SH, Bull DA, Harpole DH, et al. Outcomes after esophagectomy: a ten-year prospective cohort. Ann Thorac Surg 2003;75(1):217–22.

11. Rahimy E, Koong A, Toesca D, et al. Outcomes and tolerability of definitive and preoperative chemoradiation in elderly patients with esophageal cancer: a retro-spective institutional review. Adv Radiat Oncol 2020. https://doi.org/10.1016/j.adro.2020.05.001. S2452109420301299.

12. Yamaguchi S, Morita M, Yamamoto M, et al. Long-term outcome of definitive che-moradiotherapy and induction chemoradiotherapy followed by surgery for T4 esophageal cancer with tracheobronchial invasion. Ann Surg Oncol 2018; 25(11):3280–7.

13. Lin SH, Wang L, Myles B, et al. Propensity score-based comparison of long-term outcomes with 3-dimensional conformal radiotherapy vs intensity-modulated radiotherapy for esophageal cancer. Int J Radiat Oncol Biol Phys 2012;84(5): 1078–85.

14. van Hagen P, Hulshof MCCM, van Lanschot JJB, et al. Preoperative chemoradio-therapy for esophageal or junctional cancer. N Engl J Med 2012;366(22): 2074–84.

15. Liu S-L, Xi M, Yang H, et al. Is there a correlation between clinical complete response and pathological complete response after neoadjuvant chemoradio-therapy for esophageal squamous cell cancer? Ann Surg Oncol 2016;23(1): 273–81.

16. Toxopeus ELA, Nieboer D, Shapiro J, et al. Nomogram for predicting pathologi-cally complete response after neoadjuvant chemoradiotherapy for oesophageal cancer. Radiother Oncol 2015;115(3):392–8.

17. Noordman BJ, Shapiro J, Spaander MC, et al. Accuracy of detecting residual dis-ease after cross neoadjuvant chemoradiotherapy for esophageal cancer (pre-SANO trial): rationale and protocol. JMIR Res Protoc 2015;4(2):e79.

18. Markar S, Gronnier C, Duhamel A, et al. Salvage surgery after chemoradiother-apy in the management of esophageal cancer: is it a viable therapeutic option? J Clin Oncol 2015;33(33):3866–73.

19. Robb WB, Messager M, Dahan L, et al. Patterns of recurrence in early-stage oe-sophageal cancer after chemoradiotherapy and surgery compared with surgery alone. Br J Surg 2016;103(1):117–25.

20. Xi M, Xu C, Liao Z, et al. The impact of histology on recurrence patterns in esoph-ageal cancer treated with definitive chemoradiotherapy. Radiother Oncol 2017; 124(2):318–24.

21. Amini A, Ajani J, Komaki R, et al. Factors associated with local–regional failure after definitive chemoradiation for locally advanced esophageal cancer. Ann Surg Oncol 2014;21(1):306–14.
22. Port JL, Lee PC, Korst RJ, et al. Positron emission tomographic scanning predicts survival after induction chemotherapy for esophageal carcinoma. Ann Thorac Surg 2007;84(2):393–400.
23. Lightdale CJ, Kulkarni KG. Role of endoscopic ultrasonography in the staging and follow-up of esophageal cancer. J Clin Oncol 2005;23(20):4483–9.
24. Raymond DP, Seder CW, Wright CD, et al. Predictors of major morbidity or mortality after resection for esophageal cancer: a society of thoracic surgeons general thoracic surgery database risk adjustment model. Ann Thorac Surg 2016; 102(1):207–14.
25. Raman V, Jawitz OK, Voigt SL, et al. Surgery is associated with survival benefit in T4a esophageal adenocarcinoma: a national analysis. Ann Thorac Surg 2019; 108(6):1633–9.
26. van Ruler MAP, Peters FP, Slingerland M, et al. Clinical outcomes of definitive chemoradiotherapy using carboplatin and paclitaxel in esophageal cancer. Dis Esophagus 2017;30(4):1–9.
27. The Cancer Genome Atlas Research Network. Integrated genomic characterization of oesophageal carcinoma. Nature 2017;541(7636):169–75.
28. Bang Y-J, Van Cutsem E, Feyereislova A, et al. Trastuzumab in combination with chemotherapy versus chemotherapy alone for treatment of HER2-positive advanced gastric or gastro-oesophageal junction cancer (ToGA): a phase 3, open-label, randomised controlled trial. Lancet 2010;376(9742):687–97.
29. Fuchs CS, Doi T, Jang RW, et al. Safety and efficacy of pembrolizumab monotherapy in patients with previously treated advanced gastric and gastroesophageal junction cancer: phase 2 clinical KEYNOTE-059 trial. JAMA Oncol 2018;4(5): e180013.
30. Leichman LP, Goldman BH, Bohanes PO, et al. S0356: a phase II clinical and prospective molecular trial with oxaliplatin, fluorouracil, and external-beam radiation therapy before surgery for patients with esophageal adenocarcinoma. J Clin Oncol 2011;29(34):4555–60.

Trimodality Approach for Esophageal Malignancies

Ammara A. Watkins, MD, MPH[a], Jessica A. Zerillo, MD, MPH[b], Michael S. Kent, MD[a],*

KEYWORDS

- Trimodality therapy • Neoadjuvant • Chemoradiation • Esophageal cancer

KEY POINTS

- The standard of care for thoracic locally advanced esophageal cancer is neoadjuvant concurrent chemoradiation followed by surgery (trimodality approach).
- Definitive chemoradiation without surgery may be an option for select patients, in particular those with squamous cell histology, who have had good clinical response.
- Adjuvant nivolumab should be considered in patients who have completed trimodality therapy and have incomplete pathologic response.

INTRODUCTION

The management of locally advanced esophageal cancer has undergone significant change in the past 2 decades. Although surgical resection is a mainstay for management of locoregional esophageal cancer, 5-year survival following surgery remains poor (20%–33%).[1,2] The low cure rate following surgery alone has prompted numerous randomized controlled trials assessing the impact of chemotherapy, radiotherapy, and surgery as individual and as multimodal therapies. Trimodality therapy, the combination of neoadjuvant concurrent chemoradiation followed by surgery, has emerged as the standard of care for locoregional esophageal cancer.

DISCUSSION
Preoperative Chemoradiotherapy

Although there have been numerous trials on the topic of induction therapy for esophageal cancer, the regimens, patient populations, and results are heterogenous. Many previous trials have included gastric cancer alongside esophageal cancer at the esophagogastric junction, which complicates interpretation. Small patient size and differing patient demographics have made cumulative analysis difficult. Results of randomized trials also have been inconsistent.

[a] Division of Thoracic Surgery and Interventional Pulmonology, Department of Surgery, Beth Israel Deaconess Medical Center, Harvard Medical School, 185 Pilgrim Road, Boston, MA 02215, USA; [b] Division of Medical Oncology, Department of Medicine, Beth Israel Deaconess Medical Center, Harvard Medical School, 330 Brookline Avenue, Shapiro 9, Boston, MA 02215, USA
* Corresponding author.
E-mail address: mkent@bidmc.harvard.edu

Surg Clin N Am 101 (2021) 453–465
https://doi.org/10.1016/j.suc.2021.03.007
0039-6109/21/© 2021 Elsevier Inc. All rights reserved.

surgical.theclinics.com

In most early randomized controlled trials, no benefit for neoadjuvant chemoradiotherapy was found over surgery alone.[3–6] Several contemporary landmark trials (Radiation Therapy Oncology Group [RTOG] 85-01, Dutch CROSS [Chemotherapy for Oesophageal Cancer followed by Surgery Study], CALGB [Cancer and Leukemia Group B] 9781, and NEOCRTEC5010), however, have shown favorable results with improved long-term survival among patients receiving preoperative chemoradiation (**Table 1**).[7–9] Several meta-analyses also confirm that concurrent neoadjuvant chemoradiotherapy improves overall survival compared with any single therapy.[10–12] Neoadjuvant chemoradiation also allows patients with occult disease time to manifest disease progression. This helps avoid the morbidity of surgery, which would not be beneficial in the setting of advanced esophageal cancer. In other words, allowing for self-selection of patients who would benefit from or not benefit from surgery. Additionally, neoadjuvant chemoradiation avoids delay in systemic therapy and may improve resectability and eventual tumor margin.

Sequential Versus Concurrent Chemoradiotherapy

Data indicate that there is a survival advantage with concurrent, but not sequential, chemoradiotherapy. Three clinical trials comparing sequential chemotherapy and radiotherapy followed by surgery versus surgery alone have failed to show improvement in overall survival with the sequential trimodality group.[3,5,6] These 3 trials all included patients with squamous cell carcinoma. The earliest of these trials randomized patients to 4 treatment groups: surgery alone, preoperative chemotherapy plus surgery, preoperative radiation plus surgery, and sequential preoperative chemotherapy and radiotherapy followed by surgery.[3] Although this trial found a survival benefit in a pooled analysis among patients who received preoperative radiotherapy, there was no survival benefit found among patients who received chemotherapy, including the sequential chemoradiotherapy group.[3]

A subsequent French trial randomized patients with squamous cell carcinoma of the esophagus to preoperative sequential chemoradiation (20 Gy [Gray or radiation] and 2 courses of 5-fluorouracil and cisplatin) versus surgery alone.[6] Survival rates at 1 year and 3 years were similar between the 2 groups.[6] Another French, multicenter, randomized controlled trial comparing sequential cisplatin-based chemotherapy with 18.5 Gy of radiotherapy followed by surgery compared with surgery alone also failed to demonstrate improved survival in the sequential trimodality arm.[5] At a median follow-up of 55.2 months, no significant difference in overall survival was observed. The median survival was 18.6 months for both groups.[5] Due to these findings, concurrent chemoradiation with subsequent surgery generally is preferred for potentially resectable, T2 or higher or node-positive disease.

Neoadjuvant Chemoradiation in T2N0 Disease

The approach to clinical T2N0 esophageal cancer still is debated, with a dearth of randomized data on the topic. Most clinical trials did not stratify outcomes by histologic stage. Management differs among expert groups, with some recommending upfront surgery and others recommending induction chemoradiotherapy. For example, the NCCN recommends upfront resection if tumors are <3cm and well-differentiated.[13] In contrast, ASCO guidelines state that surgery alone may be considered if there is sufficient confidence in staging results for low-risk clinical T2N0 lesions which are well-differentiated and <2cm.[14]

The majority of retrospective literature on the topic does not show clear survival benefit for neoadjuvant treatment of clinical T2N0 disease.[15,16] Many of these studies, however, have discordant staging and are underpowered for subanalysis for

Table 1
Contemporary landmark trials for neoadjuvant chemoradiation

Trial	Tumor Types (Number of Patients)	Treatment Arms	Treatment Regimen	Median Overall Survival (mo)	5-y Overall Survival (mo)
CROSS	SCC (96)	Surgery	Carboplatin and paclitaxel (5 wk) and concurrent radiotherapy (41.4 Gy in 23 fractions, 5 d per wk) followed by esophagectomy	24	33
	Adenocarcinoma (270)	Neoadjuvant chemoradiotherapy followed by surgery		49	47
CALGB 9781	SCC (14)	Surgery	Cisplatin and fluorouracil (4 d on wk 1 and wk 5) and concurrent radiotherapy (50.4 Gy total over 5.6 wk) followed by esophagectomy	21	16
	Adenocarcinoma (42)	Neoadjuvant chemoradiotherapy		54	39
NEOCRTEC 5010	SCC (451)	Surgery	Vinorelbine (d 1 and d 8) and cisplatin (d 1–4) every 3 wk for 2 cycles and concurrent radiotherapy (40.0 Gy in 20 fractions over 5 wk) followed by esophagectomy	66.5	19
		Neoadjuvant chemoradiotherapy		100	23
RTOG 85-01	SCC (107)	Radiation	Cisplatin (first d of wk 1, 5, 8, and 11) and fluorouracil (days 1–4 on wk 1, 5, 8, and 11) with (50 Gy in 25 fractions over 5 wk)	9.3	0
	Adenocarcinoma (23)	Combined chemoradiotherapy (60 Gy)		14	26

Abbreviation: SCC, Squamous cell carcinoma.

outcomes in the understaged group.[15] Although many centers have good outcomes with upfront surgery for clinical T2N0 disease, the authors recommend neoadjuvant chemoradiation for clinical T2N0 esophageal cancer for several reasons.

First, clinical staging often is unreliable for T2N0 cancers. Studies show that upstaging of clinical T2N0 disease at time of resection is a common occurrence. Upstaging occurs in 25% to 55% of patients.[17,18] Additionally, 35% of patients are found to have nodal disease, which is linked to poor survival.[17,18] A PET scan is excellent for detecting metastasis, but it is a poor predictor of tumor size and nodal involvement. Endoscopic ultrasound (EUS), which is better suited for this assessment, still has an associated error rate. The accuracy of EUS in the detection of regional lymph nodes is 80% and 74% to 90% for the evaluation of T stage.[19] The accuracy of T stage assessment is lowest in T2 tumors, with an accuracy of 31%. Finally, contemporary trials, such as the CROSS trial, have included clinical T2N0 patients and found survival benefit with neoadjuvant chemoradiation without significant morbidity.[20]

Chemoradiotherapy Versus Surgery Alone

CROSS trial

The CROSS randomized controlled trial compared chemoradiotherapy and surgery (trimodal therapy) versus surgery alone in esophageal and esophagogastric tumors.[20] Both adenocarcinoma and squamous cell carcinoma were assessed in this trial, with squamous cell carcinoma comprising 23% of patients in each arm. The CROSS trial employed updated staging techniques, less toxic chemotherapy, and advanced radiotherapy approaches. As such, current chemoradiotherapy regimens are influenced primarily by results from the Dutch CROSS trial.[20] The CROSS regimen consisted of weekly low-dose carboplatin and paclitaxel with concurrent 41.4 Gy of radiation in 23 fractions (5 d/wk) followed by surgical resection. An R0 resection was more likely to be achieved in the trimodality group (92%) versus surgery alone group (69%; $P < .001$). Median overall survival (49.4 mo vs 24.0 mo, respectively; $P = .003$) and 5-year survival also were improved in the trimodality group (47% vs 33%, respectively; hazard ratio [HR] for death 0.67; CI, 0.51–0.87). There was a 34% lower risk of death in the follow-up period of 5 years (HR 0.657).[20]

CALGB 9781

CALGB 9781 is another randomized trial of trimodality therapy versus surgery alone among patients with stages I to III esophageal cancer. The trial initially was powered to enroll 475 patients. Due to slow accrual, however, the study was closed early and only 56 patients were enrolled (42 adenocarcinoma and 14 squamous cell carcinoma). Complete pathologic response was achieved in 40% of patients in the trimodality arm without increased morbidity or mortality compared with the surgery arm. Trimodality therapy showed a trend toward increased 5-year survival (39% vs 16%, respectively) but was not statistically significant.[8] This trial also helped establish that perioperative mortality was unchanged with the addition of preoperative chemoradiation.[8]

NEOCRTEC5010

In the Chinese NEOCRTEC5010 trial, 451 patients with esophageal squamous cell carcinoma were randomized to neoadjuvant chemoradiation (radiation concurrent with vinorelbine and cisplatin) versus surgery alone. Pathologic complete response in the chemoradiotherapy arm was 43%. Patients receiving neoadjuvant chemoradiation had a higher R0 resection rate (98% vs 91%, respectively). Median survival (100 mo vs 66.5 mo, respectively) and 3-year overall survival (69% vs 59%, respectively) also were longer in the trimodality group.[9]

Chemotherapy Versus Chemoradiotherapy

The benefit of radiation in the induction setting is not entirely clear. Radiation therapy as monotherapy no longer is recommended for curative intent based on several clinical trials and systematic reviews that have found no survival benefit.[21] A 2005 Cochrane meta-analysis reviewed 5 randomized controlled trials for a total of 1147 patients.[22] Each of the trials compared neoadjuvant radiotherapy followed by surgery to surgery alone. The overall HR was 0.89 and the meta-analysis concluded that it provided only modest survival benefit.[22] The United States Intergroup Study (INT 0123), which randomized patients to 2 different radiation doses, found that increased radiation dose was not associated with improved survival.[23] Newer radiation techniques, such as intensity-modulated radiation therapy, are beginning to be studied with hope that it also may be effective with potentially fewer side effects.

Multiple randomized trials have evaluated the benefit of neoadjuvant chemotherapy without radiation prior to surgical resection in locally advanced esophageal cancer. Five of the 7 trials demonstrated a survival benefit compared with resection alone.[1,24–27] The landmark European MAGIC (Medical Research Council Adjuvant Gastric Infusional Chemotherapy) trial demonstrated the survival benefit of perioperative chemotherapy (epirubicin, cisplatin and fluorouracil) in patients with distal esophageal, EGJ, and gastric adenocarcinoma and called into question the necessity of radiation therapy.[25] Two randomized trials directly comparing chemoradiotherapy to chemotherapy did not detect a survival advantage, but this likely was due to insufficient power.[28,29] These trials did find improved locoregional control, R0 resection rates, and complete pathologic response with chemoradiotherapy versus chemotherapy alone.[28–30] Meta-analyses, including these trials, also have concluded that R0 resections, complete pathologic response, and overall survival are improved among patients who undergo chemoradiotherapy.[3,10]

Definitive Chemoradiation

The omission of surgery is a potential option in select patients with squamous cell carcinoma histology and complete clinical response as determined by EUS and PET scan. Patients with squamous cell carcinoma have better response rates to concurrent chemoradiotherapy than patients with adenocarcinoma of the esophagus. In the CROSS regimen, 49% of patients with squamous cell carcinoma achieved complete pathologic response ($P = .008$).[20] In contrast, only 23% of patients with adenocarcinoma had a complete pathologic response.[20] Although large database analyses in the United States and Taiwan have found a survival benefit with trimodal therapy among patients with squamous cell carcinoma of the esophagus, at least 2 clinical trials have failed to see a survival benefit.[28,31–33]

In 1 trial, 172 patients were assigned to 3 cycles of induction chemotherapy with fluorouracil, leucovorin, etoposide, and cisplatin followed by concomitant chemoradiotherapy (cisplatin and etoposide with 40 Gy) and then resection, or to the same chemotherapy and chemoradiotherapy regimen followed by an additional 20 Gy of radiation therapy. Patients who had trimodality therapy had improved rates of 2-year progression-free survival (64% vs 41%, respectively) but not overall survival.[28]

In the French trial FFCD 9102, 444 patients with potentially resectable squamous cell (89%) or adenocarcinoma (11%), received induction chemotherapy with either protracted radiotherapy (46 Gy in 4.5 wk) or split course (15 Gy twice/d on days 1–5 and 22–26) schedule of concurrent radiation with chemotherapy. Patients who had a partial response and had no contraindication to surgery then were randomized to either surgery or 3 additional cycles of chemoradiotherapy (with either a 20-Gy protracted or 15-Gy split course). Two-year overall survival was not statistically significant between the 2 groups (34% vs 40%, respectively); however, surgically resected patients had lower rates of locoregional recurrence and required less palliative intervention.[31]

Currently, there are insufficient data to recommend nonsurgical management for locally advanced adenocarcinoma. There are no randomized trials directly comparing trimodality therapy with bimodal therapy. Additionally, multiple retrospective reviews indicate worse survival outcomes when surgery is omitted.[34–37] The largest retrospective analysis of patients with esophageal carcinoma treated with definitive chemoradiation is from the University of Texas MD Anderson Cancer Center.[35] This study included 215 patients with adenocarcinoma. A majority of patients had T3N1M0 disease. Approximately 98% of patients received concurrent chemoradiotherapy.[35] At a median follow-up of 54 months, 51% of patients had experienced local recurrence, 52% had distant failure with or without local recurrence, and 33% had no evidence of disease at last follow-up.[35]

Determination of what constitutes complete clinical response also is difficult. PET scan and endoscopy even with biopsy have low specificity. One retrospective analysis of patients with primarily esophageal cancer found that although 77% of patients had clinical complete response, only 31% of patients achieved pathologic complete response.[38] This inconsistency is confirmed in a systematic review and meta-analysis[39]; 44 studies were included in 1 meta-analysis. Pooled sensitivities and specificities were 33% and 95%, respectively, for endoscopic biopsies; 96% and 8%, respectively, for qualitative EUS; 74% and 52%, respectively, for qualitative PET; 89% and 72%, respectively, for PET–maximum standardized uptake value (SUVmax); and 73% and 63%, respectively, for percentage change of PET-SUVmax.[39] In a subgroup analysis, percentage change of PET-SUVmax and EUS had higher sensitivity among patients with squamous cell carcinoma than adenocarcinoma.[39]

Neoadjuvant Versus Postoperative Chemotherapy

Recovery from surgery also may affect the ability to initiate and complete adjuvant chemotherapy, even when there are no major postoperative complications. A randomized study comparing 2 different adjuvant chemotherapy regimens following resection of gastric and esophagogastric tumors found that only 60% of patients initiated adjuvant chemotherapy.[40] Similarly, in the MAGIC trial, only 54% of patients assigned to receive perioperative therapy initiated postoperative chemotherapy.[25] Reasons for not starting postoperative chemotherapy were postoperative complications, early death, patient choice, and disease progression.[25] Once adjuvant chemotherapy was initiated, a majority of patients were able to complete it. In contrast to adjuvant therapy, the preoperative CROSS regimen was well tolerated. Approximately 95% of CROSS trial participants initiated chemoradiotherapy[20]; 91% of CROSS trial participants completed chemotherapy and 92% completed prescribed radiotherapy, with few serious side effects.[20] Additionally, upfront chemotherapy allows a patient's cancer to declare its natural course. If metastasis or disease progression occurs, the patient is spared the morbidity of esophagectomy.

Preoperative chemotherapy also provides survival benefit. The Japanese trial JCOG9907 (Japan Clinical Oncology Group) compared neoadjuvant and adjuvant chemotherapy in 330 patients with clinical stage II or stage III squamous cell carcinoma of the thoracic esophagus. Patients were assigned randomly to either preoperative or postoperative chemotherapy consisting of two 21-day courses of cisplatin plus infusional fluorouracil. Five-year survival was significantly higher in the group receiving preoperative chemotherapy (55% vs 43%, respectively; $P = .04$).[41]

Cervical Esophageal Cancer

Cervical esophageal cancer accounts for 2% to 10% of esophageal cancer.[42] These cancers typically are locally advanced squamous cell carcinomas invading nearby structures, such as the airway, thyroid, and cervical lymph nodes.[42] Oncologic resection often requires radical neck dissection and resections of the pharynx, larynx, thyroid gland, and proximal esophagus. Perioperative morbidity and mortality can be as high as 50% and 10%, respectively.[43] Surgery, if performed, can be extremely morbid with no significant survival benefit over definitive chemoradiation.[43–46] Salvage esophagectomy can be considered in carefully selected patients who have persistent disease or disease recurrence for modest survival benefit (5-y survival of 17%–25% and 10-y survival of 8%).[47–49] In these scenarios, the morbidity of the operation must be balanced with the fitness of the patient, likelihood of R0 resection and small survival benefit.

A phase 2 multicenter trial assessing the efficacy of 5-fluorouracil and cisplatin–based chemotherapy with 60 Gy of radiation in 30 fractions established definitive chemoradiation as a viable option.[44] In this trial, the 3-year overall survival with chemoradiation was 66.5%.[44] The largest retrospective series, including 224 patients with cervical esophageal cancer, found that patients with a primary chemoradiotherapy approach had similar survival rates compared with the primary surgery approach. Two-year overall survival was 49.3 months for the chemoradiotherapy group and 50.7 months for the surgery group ($P > .05$).[46] Even when retrospective studies have found more modest survival rates with chemoradiation (29% at 3 y, 25% at 5 y, and 10% at 10 y); this is comparable to the 5-year overall survival with surgery alone (24%–47%).[42,50,51] Definitive chemoradiotherapy, therefore, is recommended for squamous cell carcinoma of the cervical esophagus.

HER2-positive Disease

Approximately 7% to 38% of gastroesophageal adenocarcinoma have amplification or overexpression of HER2.[52–61] Trastuzumab is a monoclonal antibody that targets HER2 and inhibits downstream signal activation and causes antibody-dependent cellular toxicity. The benefit of trastuzumab for advanced, unresectable HER2-positive adenocarcinoma of the stomach or esophagogastric junction was shown in the phase III Trastuzumab for Gastric Cancer (ToGA) trial, which compared chemotherapy with or without trastuzumab over 6 courses followed by every 3 weeks until disease progression.[56] At a median follow-up of 17 months to 19 months, median overall survival was modestly but significantly better with trastuzumab (13.8 mo vs 11.1 mo, respectively; HR 0.74; 95% CI, 0.60–0.91).[56] A phase II feasibility study for trastuzumab and pertuzumab added to neoadjuvant chemoradiation in patients with esophageal cancer also had favorable findings.[62] Patients treated with trastuzumab and pertuzumab and HER2 3+ overexpression demonstrated better survival ($P = .007$). Patients with growth factor receptor–bound protein 7–positive tumors also had better treatment response ($P = .16$).[63]

The RTOG 1010 phase III trial determined, however, that the addition of trastuzumab to trimodality therapy did not improve disease-free survival among patients with HER2 overexpressing locally advanced, resectable esophageal adenocarcinoma.[62] All patients received paclitaxel, carboplatin, and 50.4 Gy in 28 fractions. Patients were randomized 1:1 to receive weekly trastuzumab for weeks with chemoradiation and then 13 treatments every 3 weeks after surgery. The median disease-free survival time was 19.6 months for the trimodality plus trastuzumab arm compared with 14.2 months for the trimodality arm. The HR comparing the disease-free survival of trimodality plus trastuzumab arm to the trimodality arm was 0.97 (95% CI, 0.69–1.36). Median overall survival time was 38.5 months (26.2–70.4) for the trimodality plus trastuzumab arm compared with 38.9 months (29.0–64.5) for the trimodality arm (HR 1.01; 95% CI, 0.69–1.47).[62]

Targeted Therapies

Immunotherapy is a promising new treatment option in numerous solid organ malignancies, including esophageal cancer. Its use has been established in the advanced and metastatic setting. The anti–PD-1 monoclonal antibody, pembrolizumab, is approved for third-line treatment of gastric and esophagogastric junction adenocarcinoma in the United States after 2 failed chemotherapy regimens. It also is approved for locally advanced and metastatic squamous cell carcinoma of the esophagus that have high PDL-1 expression. The phase III KEYNOTE-181 trial showcased the superiority of pembrolizumab over systemic paclitaxel, docetaxel, and irinotecan.[64] This trial along with KEYNOTE-061 often are cited for off-label second-line use of pembrolizumab in patients with Siewert type I esophagogastric junction tumors.[64,65] The KEYNOTE-028 trial found favorable response with pembrolizumab in the setting of metastatic disease, particularly for adenocarcinoma.[53]

More recently, results of the CheckMate 577 trial have established nivolumab as a novel potential adjuvant treatment for patients with locally advanced esophageal and esophagogastric cancers, who have completed trimodality therapy, but have incomplete pathologic response.[66] Previously, nivolumab has been shown to be beneficial regardless of tumor cell PD-L1 expression amongst patients with advanced gastric and esophageal cancers intolerant to chemotherapy.[67,68] The CheckMate 577 trial was a global, randomized, double-blind phase III trial that assessed the effect of adjuvant nivolumab amongst patients who had stage II/III esophageal or gastroesophageal cancer, had received neoadjuvant chemoradiotherapy, had R0 resection, and had residual pathological disease. Patients who received nivolumab had significant improvement in disease-free survival with a 31% reduction in the risk of recurrence or death. The median disease-free survival was twice as long in the nivolumab group as in the placebo group (22.4 vs. 11 months).[66] The hazard ratio also favored nivolumab over placebo amongst multiple pre-specified groups including histologic type (squamous cell carcinoma and adenocarcinoma), pathological nodal status ((>ypN1and ypN0), and PD-L1 expression (<1% and >1%).[66] Based on these findings, we expect to see the addition of adjuvant nivolumab to trimodality therapy in those patients with incomplete pathologic response regardless of histology, nodal status, and PD-L1 expression.

Although the results of immunotherapy trials are encouraging, it does not yet have a role in neoadjuvant therapy for locally advanced thoracic esophageal cancer as first-line therapy. Clinical trials are currently underway analyzing the efficacy of immunotherapy on patients with locally advanced esophageal cancer in the neoadjuvant setting. Interim analysis on feasibility and safety have been promising for camrelizumab (anti-PD-1 antibody) and atezolizumab (anti-PD-L1 antibody).[69,70] A small interim analysis of 13 patients with esophagogastric and gastric cancer treated with camrelizumab and neoadjuvant FOLFOX showed 1 patient (8%) observed pathologic complete response, 3 patients (23%) achieved tumor regression, and 10 patients (77%) achieved stage reduction without any serious adverse events.[69] Clinical trials currently are under way analyzing the efficacy of immunotherapy on patients with locally advanced esophageal cancer. Interim analysis on feasibility and safety have been promising for camrelizumab (anti–PD-1 antibody) and atezolizumab (anti–PD-L1 antibody).[66,67] A small interim analysis of 13 patients with esophagogastric and gastric cancer treated with camrelizumab and neoadjuvant FOLFOX (Folinic acid, Fluorouracil, and Oxaliplatin) showed 1 patient (8%) observed pathologic complete response, 3 patients (23%) achieved tumor regression, and 10 patients (77%) achieved stage reduction without any serious adverse events.[66]

The DANTE study is phase II Study of Atezolizumab plus FLOT vs FLOT alone in patients with Gastric cancer and GEJ cancer.[67] Primary endpoints were disease progression and relapse after surgery. An interim analysis of 40 patients found only 1 patient with disease progression in the arm receiving atezolizumab, no relapse after surgery, and expected postoperative morbidity.[67] Ramucirumab (RAM), a vascular endothelial growth factor receptor type 2 (VEGF-R2) inhibitor, also has been studied in a phase II trial among patients with resectable esophagogastric adenocarcinoma treated with FLOT.[68] The addition of RAM to perioperative FLOT significantly improved R0 resection rates in the FLOT-RAM arm compared with the FLOT arm.[68] This drug has not yet been investigated among resectable thoracic esophageal cancer.

SUMMARY

Trimodality therapy is standard of care for patients with locally advanced esophageal cancer. Patients with squamous cell cancer, who have complete clinical response, may avoid surgery. Data is still accumulating about potential applications for hormonal therapy and targeted therapy for locally advanced esophageal cancer. While currently there is no role for hormonal therapy or immunotherapy in the neoadjuvant setting; there are now acceptable level 1 data for adjuvant immunotherapy for patients with locally advanced thoracic and esophagogastric esophageal cancer that have had incomplete pathologic response following trimodality therapy.

CLINICS CARE POINTS

- Trimodality therapy (concurrent chemoradiation followed by surgical resection) is the standard of care for locally advanced thoracic esophageal cancer.
- Patients with squamous cell carcinoma histology of the thoracic esophagus may be candidates for definitive chemoradiation if they have complete clinical response as determined by EUS and PET scan.
- Squamous cell carcinoma of the cervical esophagus is managed with definitive chemoradiation
- There is no role for hormonal therapy or immunotherapy in first-line treatment of locally advanced thoracic esophageal cancer; however, recent level 1 data is now available supporting adjuvant immunotherapy for patients with incomplete pathologic response following trimodality therapy.

DISCLOSURES

The authors have nothing to disclose.

REFERENCES

1. Allum WH, Stenning SP, Bancewicz J, et al. Long-term results of a randomized trial of surgery with or without preoperative chemotherapy in esophageal cancer. J Clin Oncol 2009;27:5062–7.
2. Rustgi AK, El-Serag HB. Esophageal carcinoma. N Engl J Med 2014;371: 2499–509.
3. Nygaard K, Hagen S, Hansen HS, et al. Pre-operative radiotherapy prolongs survival in operable esophageal carcinoma: a randomized, multicenter study of pre-

operative radiotherapy and chemotherapy. The second Scandinavian trial in esophageal cancer. World J Surg 1992;16:1104–9 [discussion 10].

4. Apinop C, Puttisak P, Preecha N. A prospective study of combined therapy in esophageal cancer. Hepatogastroenterology 1994;41:391–3.

5. Bosset JF, Gignoux M, Triboulet JP, et al. Chemoradiotherapy followed by surgery compared with surgery alone in squamous-cell cancer of the esophagus. N Engl J Med 1997;337:161–7.

6. Prise EL, Etienne PL, Meunier B, et al. A randomized study of chemotherapy, radiation therapy, and surgery versus surgery for localized squamous cell carcinoma of the esophagus. Cancer 1994;73:1779–84.

7. Walsh TN, Noonan N, Hollywood D, et al. A comparison of multimodal therapy and surgery for esophageal adenocarcinoma. N Engl J Med 1996;335:462–7.

8. Tepper J, Krasna MJ, Niedzwiecki D, et al. Phase III trial of trimodality therapy with cisplatin, fluorouracil, radiotherapy, and surgery compared with surgery alone for esophageal cancer: CALGB 9781. J Clin Oncol 2008;26:1086–92.

9. Yang H, Liu H, Chen Y, et al. Neoadjuvant Chemoradiotherapy followed by surgery versus surgery alone for locally advanced squamous cell carcinoma of the esophagus (NEOCRTEC5010): a phase III multicenter, randomized, open-label clinical trial. J Clin Oncol 2018;36:2796–803.

10. Chan KKW, Saluja R, Delos Santos K, et al. Neoadjuvant treatments for locally advanced, resectable esophageal cancer: A network meta-analysis. Int J Cancer 2018;143:430–7.

11. Sjoquist KM, Burmeister BH, Smithers BM, et al. Survival after neoadjuvant chemotherapy or chemoradiotherapy for resectable oesophageal carcinoma: an updated meta-analysis. Lancet Oncol 2011;12:681–92.

12. Pasquali S, Yim G, Vohra RS, et al. Survival after neoadjuvant and adjuvant treatments compared to surgery alone for resectable esophageal carcinoma: a network meta-analysis. Ann Surg 2017;265:481–91.

13. National Comprehensive Cancer Network (NCCN). NCCN clinical practice guidelines in oncology. Available at: https://www.nccn.org/professionals/physician_gls. Accessed October 6, 2020.

14. Shah M, Catenacci D, Deighton D, et al. Treatment of locally advanced esophageal cancer: ASCO guideline. J Clin Oncol 2020;38:2677–94.

15. Vining P, Birdas TJ. Management of clinical T2N0 esophageal cancer: a review. J Thorac Dis 2019;11:S1629–32.

16. Mota FC, Cecconello I, Takeda FR, et al. Neoadjuvant therapy or upfront surgery? A systematic review and meta-analysis of T2N0 esophageal cancer treatment options. Int J Surg 2018;54:176–81.

17. Markar SR, Gronnier C, Pasquer A, et al. Role of neoadjuvant treatment in clinical T2N0M0 oesophageal cancer: results from a retrospective multi-center European study. Eur J Cancer 2016;56:59–68.

18. Barbetta A, Schlottmann F, Nobel T, et al. Predictors of nodal metastases for clinical T2N0 Esophageal Adenocarcinoma. Ann Thorac Surg 2018;106:172–7.

19. Sancheti M, Fernandez F. Management of T2 esophageal cancer. Surg Clin North Am 2012;92:1169–78.

20. van Hagen P, Hulshof MC, van Lanschot JJ, et al. Preoperative chemoradiotherapy for esophageal or junctional cancer. N Engl J Med 2012;366:2074–84.

21. Cooper JS, Guo MD, Herskovic A, et al. Chemoradiotherapy of locally advanced esophageal cancer: long-term follow-up of a prospective randomized trial (RTOG 85-01). Radiation Therapy Oncology Group. JAMA 1999;281:1623–7.

22. Arnott SJ, Duncan W, Gignoux M, et al. Preoperative radiotherapy for esophageal carcinoma. Cochrane Database Syst Rev 2005;CD001799.
23. Minsky BD, Pajak TF, Ginsberg RJ, et al. INT 0123 (Radiation Therapy Oncology Group 94-05) phase III trial of combined-modality therapy for esophageal cancer: high-dose versus standard-dose radiation therapy. J Clin Oncol 2002;20:1167–74.
24. Surgical resection with or without preoperative chemotherapy in oesophageal cancer: a randomised controlled trial. The Lancet 2002;359:1727–33.
25. Cunningham D, Allum WH, Stenning SP, et al. Perioperative chemotherapy versus surgery alone for resectable gastroesophageal cancer. N Engl J Med 2006;355: 11–20.
26. Boonstra JJ, Kok TC, Wijnhoven BP, et al. Chemotherapy followed by surgery versus surgery alone in patients with resectable oesophageal squamous cell carcinoma: long-term results of a randomized controlled trial. BMC Cancer 2011;11:181.
27. Ychou M, Boige V, Pignon JP, et al. Perioperative chemotherapy compared with surgery alone for resectable gastroesophageal adenocarcinoma: an FNCLCC and FFCD multicenter phase III trial. J Clin Oncol 2011;29:1715–21.
28. Stahl M, Walz MK, Stuschke M, et al. Phase III comparison of preoperative chemotherapy compared with chemoradiotherapy in patients with locally advanced adenocarcinoma of the esophagogastric junction. J Clin Oncol 2009; 27:851–6.
29. Burmeister BH, Thomas JM, Burmeister EA, et al. Is concurrent radiation therapy required in patients receiving preoperative chemotherapy for adenocarcinoma of the oesophagus? A randomised phase II trial. Eur J Cancer 2011;47:354–60.
30. Klevebro F, Alexandersson von Dobeln G, Wang N, et al. A randomized clinical trial of neoadjuvant chemotherapy versus neoadjuvant chemoradiotherapy for cancer of the oesophagus or gastro-oesophageal junction. Ann Oncol 2016;27:660–7.
31. Bedenne L, Michel P, Bouche O, et al. Chemoradiation followed by surgery compared with chemoradiation alone in squamous cancer of the esophagus: FFCD 9102. J Clin Oncol 2007;25:1160–8.
32. Naik KB, Liu Y, Goodman M, et al. Concurrent chemoradiotherapy with or without surgery for patients with resectable esophageal cancer: an analysis of the National Cancer Data Base. Cancer 2017;123:3476–85.
33. McKenzie S, Mailey B, Artinyan A, et al. Improved outcomes in the management of esophageal cancer with the addition of surgical resection to chemoradiation therapy. Ann Surg Oncol 2011;18:551–8.
34. Tougeron D, Scotte M, Hamidou H, et al. Definitive chemoradiotherapy in patients with esophageal adenocarcinoma: an alternative to surgery? J Surg Oncol 2012; 105:761–6.
35. Sudo K, Xiao L, Wadhwa R, et al. Importance of surveillance and success of salvage strategies after definitive chemoradiation in patients with esophageal cancer. J Clin Oncol 2014;32:3400–5.
36. Shridhar R, Freilich J, Hoffe SE, et al. Single-institution retrospective comparison of preoperative versus definitive chemoradiotherapy for adenocarcinoma of the esophagus. Ann Surg Oncol 2014;21:3744–50.
37. Goense L, van Rossum PSN, Xi M, et al. Preoperative nomogram to risk stratify patients for the benefit of trimodality therapy in esophageal adenocarcinoma. Ann Surg Oncol 2018;25:1598–607.
38. Cheedella NK, Suzuki A, Xiao L, et al. Association between clinical complete response and pathological complete response after preoperative chemoradiation in patients with gastroesophageal cancer: analysis in a large cohort. Ann Oncol 2013;24:1262–6.

39. Eyck BM, Onstenk BD, Noordman BJ, et al. Accuracy of detecting residual disease after neoadjuvant chemoradiotherapy for esophageal cancer: a systematic review and meta-analysis. Ann Surg 2020;271:245–56.
40. Al-Batran S-E, Homann N, Pauligk C, et al. Perioperative chemotherapy with fluorouracil plus leucovorin, oxaliplatin, and docetaxel versus fluorouracil or capecitabine plus cisplatin and epirubicin for locally advanced, resectable gastric or gastro-oesophageal junction adenocarcinoma (FLOT4): a randomised, phase 2/3 trial. The Lancet 2019;393:1948–57.
41. Ando N, Kato H, Igaki H, et al. A randomized trial comparing postoperative adjuvant chemotherapy with cisplatin and 5-fluorouracil versus preoperative chemotherapy for localized advanced squamous cell carcinoma of the thoracic esophagus (JCOG9907). Ann Surg Oncol 2012;19:68–74.
42. Hoeben A, Polak J, Van De Voorde L, et al. Cervical esophageal cancer: a gap in cancer knowledge. Ann Oncol 2016;27:1664–74.
43. Valmasoni M, Pierobon ES, Zanchettin G, et al. Cervical esophageal cancer treatment strategies: a cohort study appraising the debated role of surgery. Ann Surg Oncol 2018;25:2747–55.
44. Zenda S, Kojima T, Kato K, et al. Multicenter Phase 2 Study of Cisplatin and 5-Fluorouracil with concurrent radiation therapy as an organ preservation approach in patients with squamous cell carcinoma of the cervical esophagus. Int J Radiat Oncol Biol Phys 2016;96:976–84.
45. Zhang P, Xi M, Zhao L, et al. Clinical efficacy and failure pattern in patients with cervical esophageal cancer treated with definitive chemoradiotherapy. Radiother Oncol 2015;116:257–61.
46. Cao CN, Luo JW, Gao L, et al. Primary radiotherapy compared with primary surgery in cervical esophageal cancer. JAMA Otolaryngol Head Neck Surg 2014; 140:918–26.
47. Schieman C, Wigle DA, Deschamps C, et al. Salvage resections for recurrent or persistent cancer of the proximal esophagus after chemoradiotherapy. Ann Thorac Surg 2013;95:459–63.
48. Gardner-Thorpe J, Hardwick RH, Dwerryhouse SJ. Salvage oesophagectomy after local failure of definitive chemoradiotherapy. Br J Surg 2007;94:1059–66.
49. Kumagai K, Mariosa D, Tsai JA, et al. Systematic review and meta-analysis on the significance of salvage esophagectomy for persistent or recurrent esophageal squamous cell carcinoma after definitive chemoradiotherapy. Dis Esophagus 2016;29:734–9.
50. Gkika E, Gauler T, Eberhardt W, et al. Long-term results of definitive radiochemotherapy in locally advanced cancers of the cervical esophagus. Dis Esophagus 2014;27:678–84.
51. Daiko H, Hayashi R, Saikawa M, et al. Surgical management of carcinoma of the cervical esophagus. J Surg Oncol 2007;96:166–72.
52. Park YS, Hwang HS, Park HJ, et al. Comprehensive analysis of HER2 expression and gene amplification in gastric cancers using immunohistochemistry and in situ hybridization: which scoring system should we use? Hum Pathol 2012;43:413–22.
53. Doi T, Piha-Paul SA, Jalal SI, et al. Safety and antitumor activity of the anti-programmed death-1 antibody pembrolizumab in patients with advanced esophageal carcinoma. J Clin Oncol 2018;36:61–7.
54. Barros-Silva JD, Leitao D, Afonso L, et al. Association of ERBB2 gene status with histopathological parameters and disease-specific survival in gastric carcinoma patients. Br J Cancer 2009;100:487–93.

55. Liang Z, Zeng X, Gao J, et al. Analysis of EGFR, HER2, and TOP2A gene status and chromosomal polysomy in gastric adenocarcinoma from Chinese patients. BMC Cancer 2008;8:363.
56. Bang Y-J, Van Cutsem E, Feyereislova A, et al. Trastuzumab in combination with chemotherapy versus chemotherapy alone for treatment of HER2-positive advanced gastric or gastro-oesophageal junction cancer (ToGA): a phase 3, open-label, randomised controlled trial. The Lancet 2010;376:687–97.
57. Kim KC, Koh YW, Chang HM, et al. Evaluation of HER2 protein expression in gastric carcinomas: comparative analysis of 1,414 cases of whole-tissue sections and 595 cases of tissue microarrays. Ann Surg Oncol 2011;18:2833–40.
58. Koopman T, Smits MM, Louwen M, et al. HER2 positivity in gastric and esopha-geal adenocarcinoma: clinicopathological analysis and comparison. J Cancer Res Clin Oncol 2015;141:1343–51.
59. Tanner M, Hollmen M, Junttila TT, et al. Amplification of HER-2 in gastric carci-noma: association with Topoisomerase IIalpha gene amplification, intestinal type, poor prognosis and sensitivity to trastuzumab. Ann Oncol 2005;16:273–8.
60. Gravalos C, Jimeno A. HER2 in gastric cancer: a new prognostic factor and a novel therapeutic target. Ann Oncol 2008;19:1523–9.
61. Fornaro L, Vivaldi C, Parnofiello A, et al. Validated clinico-pathologic nomogram in the prediction of HER2 status in gastro-oesophageal cancer. Br J Cancer 2019; 120:522–6.
62. Safran H, Winter KA, Wigle DA, et al. Trastuzumab with trimodality treatment for esophageal adenocarcinoma with HER2 overexpression: NRG Oncology/RTOG 1010. J Clin Oncol 2020;38:4500.
63. Stroes CI, Schokker S, Creemers A, et al. Phase II feasibility and biomarker study of neoadjuvant trastuzumab and pertuzumab with chemoradiotherapy for resect-able human epidermal growth factor receptor 2-positive esophageal adenocarci-noma: TRAP Study. J Clin Oncol 2020;38:462–71.
64. Kim SB, Doi T, Kato K, et al. KEYNOTE-181: Pembrolizumab vs chemotherapy in patients (pts) with advanced/metastatic adenocarcinoma (AC) or squamous cell carcinoma (SCC) of the esophagus as second-line (2L) therapy. Ann Oncol 2019; 30:ix42–3.
65. Alsina M, Moehler M, Lorenzen S. Immunotherapy of esophageal cancer: current status, many trials and innovative strategies. Oncol Res Treat 2018;41:266–71.
66. Kelly RJ, Ajani JA, Kuzdzal J, et al. Adjuvant Nivolumab in Resected Esophageal or Gastroesophageal Junction Cancer. N Engl J Med 2021;384:1191–203.
67. Boku N, Satoh T, Ryu MH, et al. Nivolumab in previously treated advanced gastric cancer (ATTRACTION-2): 3-year update and outcome of treatment beyond pro-gression with nivolumab. Gastric Cancer 2021.
68. Kato K, Cho BC, Takahashi M, et al. Nivolumab versus chemotherapy in patients with advanced oesophageal squamous cell carcinoma refractory or intolerant to previous chemotherapy (ATTRACTION-3): a multicentre, randomised, open-la-bel, phase 3 trial. The Lancet Oncology 2019;20:1506–17.
69. Liu Y, Han G, Li H, et al. Camrelizumab combined with FOLFOX as neoadjuvant therapy for resectable locally advanced gastric and gastroesophageal junction adenocarcinoma. Journal of Clinical Oncology 2020;38:4536.
70. Al-Batran S-E, Lorenzen S, Schenk M, et al. Safety of perioperative atezolizumab in combination with FLOT versus FLOT alone in patients with resectable esopha-gogastric adenocarcinoma: An interim safety analysis of the DANTE, a random-ized, open-label phase II trial of the German Gastric Group at the AIO and the SAKK. Journal of Clinical Oncology 2020;38:398.

Salvage Esophagectomy

Romulo Fajardo, MD[a], Abbas E. Abbas, MD, MS[b],
Roman V. Petrov, MD, PhD[b], Charles T. Bakhos, MD, MS[b],*

KEYWORDS

- Chemoradiation • Delayed esophagectomy • Planned resection • Outcomes
- Neoadjuvant

KEY POINTS

- Salvage esophagectomy can be offered after definitive chemoradiation therapy (CRT) or in the setting of active surveillance after neoadjuvant CRT.
- Although salvage resection offers patients with locally advanced esophageal cancer a chance at improved long-term survival, it is associated with higher morbidity compared with planned esophagectomy.
- Special technical considerations must be taken into account when considering salvage esophagectomy, such as radiation dose, radiation field, conduit of choice, and tumor location.
- In order to optimize outcomes and minimize morbidity, salvage esophagectomy should be considered in a multidisciplinary setting involving experienced high-volume surgeons.

INTRODUCTION

Esophageal cancer is the sixth leading cause of cancer-related deaths worldwide.[1,2] Despite advancements in neoadjuvant and adjuvant treatment modalities, as well as the advent of minimally invasive surgical approaches, the overall 5-year survival rate in the United States remains approximately 19.9% (Esophageal Cancer—Cancer Stat Facts, DOI: 08/21/20). Although multiple studies have demonstrated the survival benefit of neo-adjuvant chemoradiation followed by esophagectomy,[3–6] other randomized trials did not show a clear survival benefit of surgery after chemoradiation treatment (CRT) in esophageal squamous cell carcinoma (ESCC).[7–9] This led to question the value of added surgery to chemoradiation in the management of locoregional esophageal cancer.[10] In this setting, salvage esophagectomy can be offered for patients who fail chemoradiation and have evidence of locoregional recurrence or persistent disease. Additionally, salvage esophagectomy can be offered for patients who underwent induction chemoradiation but did not or could not undergo surgery in a timely manner, because of worsening functional status or other medical or nonmedical reasons.

[a] Department of Surgery, Temple University Hospital, 3401 North Broad Street C-401, Philadelphia, PA 19140, USA; [b] Lewis Katz School of Medicine at Temple University, Temple University Hospital, 3401 North Broad Street C-501, Philadelphia, PA 19140, USA
* Corresponding author.
E-mail address: Charles.Bakhos@tuhs.temple.edu

Surg Clin N Am 101 (2021) 467–482
https://doi.org/10.1016/j.suc.2021.03.008
0039-6109/21/© 2021 Elsevier Inc. All rights reserved.

   This article reviews the indications and outcomes of salvage esophagectomy and discusses its role in the management of locally advanced esophageal cancer.

PATIENT SELECTION AND EVALUATION

The first category of patients who would be eligible for a salvage esophagectomy is those who undergo definitive CRT for locally advanced esophageal cancer and have either persistent or recurrent disease. The second category is patients who undergo induction CRT regimens followed by active surveillance of locoregional relapse or persistent disease. This wait and watch treatment pathway (**Fig. 1**) would allow

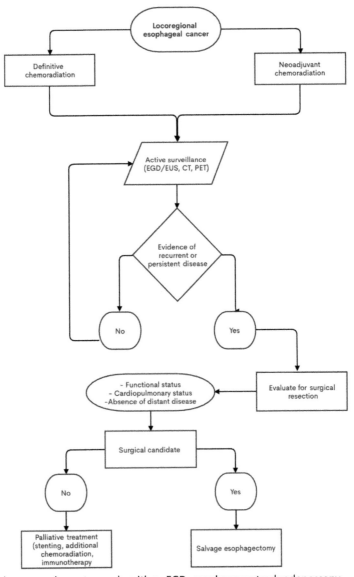

Fig. 1. Salvage esophagectomy algorithm. EGD, esophagogastroduodenoscopy.

organ preservation and more selective resection, thereby avoiding the morbidity of esophagectomy, especially in those patients who show evidence of complete pathologic response after CRT.[11] Finally, some patients undergo delayed esophagectomy after induction chemoradiation, because they could not proceed with their planned surgery because of deterioration of their functional status or other reasons. There is no clear definition of delayed esophagectomy in the literature, and the distinction between salvage surgery can be blurred. In general, though, surgical resection is considered delayed if it occurs more than 3 months from the end of CRT.

Along with the review of these categories of patients, other important factors that are discussed include, among others, the underlying histology (adenocarcinoma vs squamous cell carcinoma), location of the tumor (ie, peritracheal vs distal esophageal), and the difference in radiation dosage.

SALVAGE ESOPHAGECTOMY AFTER DEFINITIVE CHEMORADIATION TREATMENT

Definitive chemoradiation without intended resection is the standard of treatment of patients with unfavorable tumor location (cervical esophagus), with unresectable tumors (cT4b), and who are too frail or who simply decline surgical therapy.[12] Historically, the Radiation Therapy Oncology Group (RTOG) 85-01 study showed superiority of concurrent chemoradiation over radiotherapy alone in a randomized trial of 129 patients with locally advanced resectable esophageal cancer (82.3% squamous cell carcinoma [ESCC] and 17.7% adenocarcinoma). This study showed the ability to achieve prolonged survival with nonsurgical therapy; however, there were a significant number of patients (56%) who failed locoregional control.[13] The 5-year overall survival rates with combined treatment versus radiation therapy alone were 26% and 0%, respectively. There was no significant difference in survival related to histologic tumor type for patients treated with combined therapy. Combined therapy consisted of 50 Gy given over 5 weeks with combined fluorouracil-cisplatin therapy as opposed to radiation therapy alone, which was given at a higher dose, of 64 Gy, over 6.4 weeks. The trial confirmed the survival benefit of CRT over radiation therapy alone, but the effects of combined therapy may have been underestimated due to using a smaller radiation dose.

Consequently, the RTOG 94-05 was designed to evaluate the use of higher levels of radiation (64.8 Gy) to decrease locoregional recurrence in the treatment field.[14] The trial failed to show, however, improved locoregional control or survival and was stopped after interim analysis. Minsky and colleagues[14] concluded that a radiation dose of 50 Gy (dosage originally used in the RTOG 85-01 trial) be used as the standard definitive dose for definitive CRT for thoracic esophageal carcinoma. Furthermore, and because of the higher morbidity and complication rate associated with higher doses of radiation, 41.4 Gy is advocated by many centers as the preferred regimen in the neoadjuvant setting.[6,15]

Because esophagectomy carries a significant risk of mortality and morbidity, and, because surgically unfit patients would opt for medical treatment with limited success, clinicians started to investigate the use of definitive CRT in patients with better performance status and resectable disease. In that regard, several randomized controlled trials reported the short-term and long-term outcomes with nonsurgical therapy.[7,9,13,14] In the FFCD 9102 trial, which compared definitive CRT (total 66 Gy) versus chemoradiation (total 46 Gy) followed by surgery for ESCC (88.8%) and adenocarcinoma (11.2%), Bedenne and colleagues[7] reported a 2-year survival rate of 34% in the surgical arm and 40% in the definitive CRT-only arm ($P = .44$). The 2-year local control rates were 66.4% versus 57% in their surgical versus CRT arms, respectively.

The 3-month mortality rate, however, was significantly higher in the surgical arm in comparison with CRT only (9.3% vs 0.8%, respectively; P<.001). The investigators concluded that in patients with locally advanced esophageal cancers who respond to chemoradiation, there is no benefit for the addition of surgery after chemoradiation compared with definitive CRT.

Similarly, Stahl and colleagues[9] conducted a randomized trial comparing chemoradiation (40 Gy) followed by surgery versus definitive CRT alone (>65 Gy) for ESCC; in contrast to the Bedenne and colleagues'[7] trial, however, all patients were randomized and not just the responders. The investigators showed that locoregional recurrence was higher in the definitive CRT group and that the 2-year disease-free survival was significantly higher in the surgical group compared with definitive CRT (64% vs 41%, respectively; P = .0003). Not surprisingly, there was a significantly higher treatment-related mortality reported in the surgical arm (12.8% vs 3.5%, respectively; P = .03). This highlights the fact that patients who underwent surgery were more likely to experience treatment-related mortality and morbidity than die from the cancer itself. Noteworthy in this study is that nonresponders who achieved an R0 resection had a 3-year survival rate of 32%, compared with those with tumor response who achieved greater than 50% 3-year survival.[9]

These 2 studies demonstrated that in patients who respond to definitive CRT, the risk of surgery-related complications or toxicity may offset the potential increase in survival conferred by resection and that nonresponders may benefit more from the addition of surgery.

In this setting, salvage esophagectomy after definitive CRT is a viable option for patients who develop recurrent or persistent disease without evidence of distant metastases. There are many prospective, nonrandomized, and retrospective studies that describe the feasibility of salvage resection mostly in patients with ESCC but also for esophageal adenocarcinoma.[16–28] In 2012, Marks and colleagues[23] compared outcomes of salvage resection after failed definitive CRT to matched patients who underwent induction CRT and planned resection for esophageal adenocarcinoma. Differences in radiation dose were accounted for in the matched-pair analysis (approximately 45 Gy); 30-day mortality, 3-year overall survival, and median survival rates between the 2 groups were not statistically different (n = 65 in each arm). The investigators concluded that postoperative mortality and morbidity after salvage esophagectomy are comparable to matched patients after planned resection, suggesting that patients with esophageal adenocarcinoma who fail definitive CRT and have locoregional recurrence should be considered for salvage resection at experienced high-volume centers.

Tachimori and colleagues[24] reviewed 59 consecutive patients with ESCC who underwent salvage resection for locoregional failure after definitive CRT (>60 Gy). Postoperative morbidity and mortality rates were higher among patients who underwent salvage esophagectomy compared with those who underwent resection without preoperative CRT (hospital mortality rates, 8% vs 2%, respectively). Three-year postoperative survival rates for salvage resection versus resection without preoperative CRT were 38% versus 58%, respectively. The investigators concluded that although salvage resection has increased rates of morbidity and mortality, salvage esophagectomy could provide long-term survival and should be considered for carefully selected patients at specialized centers.[24]

In the authors' practice, the timing of diagnosis is taken into consideration to differentiate treatment failures further after definitive CRT. When a "recurrence" is noted within a few months of CRT, this most likely is persistent disease and possibly is a poor prognosticator for long-term survival in this group of patients. Such patients have only palliative systemic therapy as an alternative to surgery. On the other hand, when a true local recurrence is noted many months or years after CRT, such patients may be expected to have better overall outcomes.

SALVAGE ESOPHAGECTOMY AFTER INDUCTION CHEMORADIATION TREATMENT

For those patients with locally advanced esophageal cancer who undergo induction chemoradiation therapy (CRT), a strategy of active surveillance and watchful waiting has been proposed in an organ preservation effort and to avoid the morbidity of esophagectomy. This also has been justified by the non-negligible proportion of patients who exhibit evidence of full pathologic response after CRT. For instance, 29% (47 of 161) of patients with esophageal cancer showed a pathologically complete response after receiving neoadjuvant chemoradiation followed by resection in the CROSS trial using the regimen of carboplatin, paclitaxel, and concurrent 41.4-Gy radiotherapy.[5] Although a complete pathologic response was seen in 49% (18 of 37) of patients with squamous cell carcinoma and 23% (28 of 121) with adenocarcinoma ($P = .008$), histologic tumor cell type was not a prognostic factor for improved survival. The MAGIC trial, which compared outcomes between perioperative chemotherapy followed by surgery versus surgery alone for resectable esophageal, esophagogastric, or gastric adenocarcinoma, found a higher rate of pathologic response (tumor shrinkage, less advanced tumor stage, and nodal involvement) in patients who underwent perioperative chemotherapy versus surgery alone.[29] Among all patients with adenocarcinoma who underwent resection, 51.7% of those in the perioperative-chemotherapy group combined with surgery had a less advanced tumor stage (T1 and T2 tumors) as opposed to only 36.8% of those in the surgery-alone group ($P = .002$). Because an accurate pathologic response evaluation requires surgical resection, clinicians have in practice to rely on clinical response evaluation. In that regard, Taketa and colleagues[30] retrospectively reviewed 622 patients after chemoradiation and surgery (93.5% adenocarcinoma); 61 patients were considered to have complete clinical response after neoadjuvant CRT as confirmed by endoscopic tumor cell biopsies and PET–computed tomography (CT) and refused surgery. These patients showed a 5-year overall and recurrence-free survival of 58.1% and 35.3% respectively. Using propensity-score matching, no difference in 3-year overall survival was found between the patients who declined surgery and those who underwent the standard trimodality therapy (62% vs 56%, respectively; $P = .28$).[30]

Castoro and colleagues[31] compared outcomes of patients who achieved a complete clinical response to neoadjuvant CRT (45–50 Gy) plus esophagectomy to those patients who had a complete clinical response without surgery. This study included 77 patients with squamous cell carcinoma of the esophagus (39 patients in surgical arm and 38 patients in the nonsurgical arm). Differences in 5-year overall survival and disease-free survival were not statistically significant ($P = .99$ and $P = .15$, respectively), even with adjusting for propensity score, age, American Society of Anesthesiologists score, and clinical stage ($P = .65$ and $P = .15$, respectively). The investigators concluded that a wait and watch approach for using salvage esophageal resection did not negatively affect survival.[31]

A key component to the active surveillance strategy for managing locally advanced esophageal cancer is the degree at which patients achieve clinical response to CRT. To prevent the occurrence of nonresectable recurrent disease, residual disease should be detected accurately at an early stage. There is no standardized protocol for evaluating clinical responses in patients receiving neoadjuvant CRT, and most evaluation protocols involve endoscopy with biopsy, endoscopic ultrasonography (EUS), PET, CT, and magnetic resonance imaging (MRI). These surveillance modalities are discussed Bakhos C, Acevedo E, Petrov R, Abbas A. Surveillance following treatment for esophageal cancer, in this issue.

DELAYED ESOPHAGECTOMY

For patients undergoing trimodality therapy for locally advanced esophageal adeno-carcinoma, CRT followed by surgery 4 weeks to 6 weeks later is the standard timing for resection.[5,6] Timing of appropriate resection may not always be feasible due to factors, such as patient preference, comorbidities, poor functional status after CRT, and lack of surgical consultation. This may result in a greater time lapse between the end of CRT to timely resection. As discussed previously, there is no clear definition delayed esophagectomy in the literature, but, in general, surgical resection that occurs more than 3 months after the end of neoadjuvant therapy is considered as such. Delayed and salvage esophagectomy are not exactly the same, but both historically have been associated with increased pulmonary complications and perioperative mortality.[16–18,32,33] Other reports, however, showed similar morbidity and overall survival.[23,34–36] More recently, Levinsky and colleagues[37] sought out to evaluate the outcomes for delayed and salvage esophagectomy for esophageal adeno-carcinoma. The investigators analyzed 8489 patients in the National Cancer Database between 2004 and 2014 for patients with clinical stage II and stage III esophageal adenocarcinoma who underwent preoperative CRT and esophagectomy. Patients were divided into 2 groups, those who underwent resection less than 90 days (n = 7822) and those who had surgery >90 days (n = 667) after completion of CRT. They found that delayed esophagectomy was associated with higher rates of pathologic complete response (22.2% vs 18.6%, respectively; P = .043) and 90-day postoperative mortality (10.4% vs 7.8%, respectively; $P<.01$). On multivariate analysis, however, delayed esophagectomy was not independently associated with decreased overall survival. Levinksy and colleagues[37] concluded that delayed and salvage esophagectomy may be offered to patients who did not receive timely surgical resection after CRT.

TECHNICAL CONSIDERATIONS

Salvage resection should be performed in the same manner as a standard esophagectomy, including the use of minimally invasive techniques, depending on surgeon experience. Example photos of port placement can be seen in **Figs. 2** and **3**. There are a

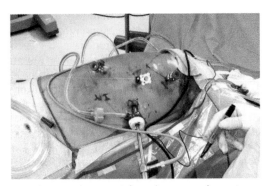

Fig. 2. Robotic thorascopic port placement for salvage esophagectomy.

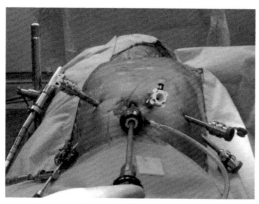

Fig. 3. Robotic laparoscopic port placement for salvage esophagectomy.

few points to consider, however, when performing esophagectomy in the salvage setting, mainly the radiation dosage and treatment field and their potential impact on the health of the conduit.[16,38]

For instance, a recent systematic and meta-analysis reported a rate of conduit necrosis in salvage esophagectomy as high as 21%,[39] with a mortality rate reaching 90% in another report.[40] Risk factors associated with conduit ischemia or necrosis include diabetes mellitus, malnutrition, steroid use, hypertension, cardiac arrhythmias, reduced cardiac contractility, and peripheral vascular disease.[41] Irradiation of the esophagus and stomach, especially for lower esophageal tumors and/or higher radiation dosages, may negatively affect the conduit microvasculature and perfusion, thus contributing to leakage.[24,35] Although the stomach is the most commonly used conduit for its robust blood supply and technical feasibility for being an esophageal replacement (**Table 1**), special attention must be paid to the radiation treatment plan and if the entire stomach was included in the treatment field. Intraoperative careful examination of the stomach should be performed for signs of injury or unsuitability for conduit reconstruction. Intraoperative assessment of conduit perfusion as it pertains to color, viability, and degree of anastomotic edge bleeding is subjective, therefore may not be objectively accurate.[41] More advanced and objective measures to assess conduit perfusion have been developed to guide intraoperative assessment, which include fluorescence angiography, laser doppler flowmetry and spectrophotometry, and laser-induced fluorescence of indocyanine green (ICG).[42–55] Ohi and colleagues[49] conducted a retrospective analysis investigating the impact of ICG fluorescein imaging of the gastric conduit during esophagectomy. Univariate analysis showed an increased risk of anastomotic leakage in patients who did not undergo ICG fluorescein imaging ($P = .0057$), and multivariate analysis revealed that the absence of ICG imaging was an independent risk factor for the development of an anastomotic leak ($P = .05$). Other studies, however, did not demonstrate the benefits of robotic Firefly (Da Vinci Vision, Intuitive Surgical, Sunnyvale, CA, USA) and ICG.[52,56,57] Further randomized trials specifically looking at the use of ICG assessment and other modalities during esophagectomy still are required.

Additionally, placing the anastomosis within the radiated field in the chest has been associated with an increased leak rate,[58] and for this reason it generally is preferable to have the anastomosis above it whenever possible.[59] When there is concern for the viability of the esophageal conduit, options include transposition of an omental harvest along the suture or staple line, consideration for the use of a different conduit, such as

Table 1
Esophageal replacement conduit options

	Advantages	Disadvantages	Pearls
Stomach[74,75]	• Sufficient length • Predictable and robust vascular supply • Requires single anastomosis	• Common site for previous surgeries (sacrificed right gastroepiploic artery) • May be included in radiation field	• Preservation of right gastroepiploic • Most commonly used esophageal substitute
Colon[76–79]	• Substantial length • Acid resistance • Choice of right or left colon (both include transverse colon)	• Susceptible to native common pathology • Loss of absorptive capacity • May lengthen over time • Requires microvascular technique for supercharging • Requires multiple anastomoses • May present a size mismatch between native esophagus	• Mobilization of entire colon to assess vascular anatomy • Supercharging and/or super-drainage may be required for inadequate arterial or venous supply respectively • CT angiogram may assist in operative planning • Colonoscopy or double barium enema should be obtained to rule primary colonic pathology • Preoperative clear liquid diet and bowel preparation
Jejunum[74,75]	• Significant amount of redundant jejunum • Predictable and reliable blood supply • Usually lacks intrinsic pathology • Has intrinsic peristalsis • Does not undergo senescent lengthening • Similar caliber to native esophagus	• Fatty mesentery may hinder positioning • May not have adequate length for cervical anastomosis • Requires microvascular technique for supercharging • Requires multiple anastomoses	• Mesentery must be divided to straighten and reduce redundancy of the conduit • Supercharging and/or super-drainage is an option • CT angiogram may assist operative planning

the colon or long segment jejunum. Sepesi and colleagues[60] evaluated the use of thoracic transposition of an omental flap along the gastric conduit to reduce the incidence of anastomotic leak or need for reoperation after esophagectomy. Patients with an omental flap had significantly lower rate of anastomotic leakage in comparison to those without (4.7% vs 10.5%, respectively; $P = .014$). Reoperations to salvage the gastric conduit were less common with those patients who had an omental flap transposition ($P = .024$). They concluded that the use of a pedicled omental transposition flap to reinforce all thoracic anastomoses is recommended.

Another important factor to consider is tumor location in respect to the trachea. Booka and colleagues[61] found that patients with upper thoracic esophageal tumors were more likely to undergo incomplete resection ($P = .011$), due to the positive radial margin invading into the trachea. Furthermore, the close proximity of the trachea to the esophagus, especially in an irradiated field, may be associated with a higher risk of tracheoesophageal fistula in patients undergoing salvage esophagectomy. Planned resection often is advocated for these patients as bimodal therapy and a selective approach may render the tumor unresectable.[11]

If there is any doubt of conduit viability or suspicion for conduit ischemia intraoperatively, a delayed reconstruction approach should be initiated using colon or small bowel. In 2009, Oezcelik and colleagues[62] reported a series of 554 patients who underwent esophagectomy with gastric pullup. In 37 patients (7%), graft ischemia along with significant comorbidities resulted in delayed neck anastomosis. The gastric conduit was brought up and secured in the neck and a cervical esophagostomy was performed. A delayed esophagogastric anastomosis (median of 22 months) was performed and 0% of patients developed conduit ischemia or necrosis.

When colon is used as a conduit in nonsalvage resections, graft necrosis has been reported as high as 16%.[63] This may be due to bacterial contamination, especially if the patient has not been prepped preoperatively. The technique of a supercharged colonic interposition graft as an adjunct to esophagocolonic anastomosis has been described to reduce the morbidity of ischemic-related complications.[64,65] This technique requires microvascular anastomoses in the neck to augment venous drainage and arterial supply to the colonic graft. Fujita and colleagues[64] compared 24 patients who underwent reconstruction without supercharged colonic interposition to 29 patients with supercharged colon. They showed that the group of patients who received supercharged colonic interposition grafts had a significantly lower rate of conduit necrosis and anastomotic leakage (7% vs 54%; $P = .0002$).[64]

Jejunal reconstruction has some technical advantages, including the relative ease in mobilizing a long segment of jejunum and sizable mesenteric blood vessels (see **Table 1**). Disadvantages include that it is a rare form of esophageal replacement and is performed only at high-volume experienced centers. Supercharged jejunal conduits also has been described with relative success.[66] Contraindications for performing jejunal esophageal replacement include Crohn disease, short bowel syndrome, and short fatty mesentery. Jejunal conduit necrosis usually occurs due to technical errors, poor vascular supply, venous thrombosis, and perioperative hypotension.[67] Ascioti and colleagues[68] retrospectively reviewed 26 patients who had undergone reconstruction with supercharged jejunum and found a cervical anastomotic rate of 19.2%, a 7.7% rate of conduit loss, and 0% mortality. These different conduit options are listed in **Table 1**.

The authors' approach is to tackle all esophagectomies, including delayed and salvage procedures using the robotic platform. This allows excellent determination of resectability and better tissue handling thanks to the motion-scaled wristed instruments. This is important especially when dissecting the esophagus off the airway because often radiation-induced fibrosis may make this dissection particularly difficult and hazardous. The authors also routinely employ in such cases ICG autofluorescence in order to assess the tissue perfusion of the conduit, which may be compromised secondary to the long-term effects of radiation on the vasculature.

ENDOSCOPIC SALVAGE RESECTION

Although salvage esophagectomy is the treatment of choice for locoregional recurrence after definitive or neoadjuvant CRT, endoscopic therapy or tumor enucleation with minimally invasive hybrid techniques may be considered for those who elect not to undergo salvage resection or have physical conditions precluding an invasive procedure. Local tumor recurrence depth evaluated by EUS is critical in determining this treatment modality. There are a few reports in the literature describing endoscopic mucosal resection (EMR) in the salvage setting. Makazu and colleagues[69] retrospectively reviewed 11 patients (13 lesions) with local recurrence (9/11) or residual (2/11) tumor who underwent salvage EMR. The depth of tumor resection was limited to the mucosal layer in 7 lesions and submucosal in the remaining 6 lesions. En bloc resection was performed on 6 lesions and the vertical margin was free of disease in 11 lesions (84.6%). No major complications were observed. At median follow-up of 38.9 months following salvage EMR, no recurrence was detected in 6 patients (54%). The 5-year survival rate after salvage EMR was 41.6%. Albeit a single case report, another interesting approach for salvage treatment has been described, consisting of a minimally invasive hybrid enucleation for local recurrence in a single patient with recurrence confined to the esophageal muscular layer.[70]

OUTCOMES OF SALVAGE ESOPHAGECTOMY

The main goal of esophagectomy is to eradicate esophageal cancer. This is true especially in the salvage setting, where patients have evidence of persistent or recurrent disease after chemoradiation, and surgical resection representing their last chance of cure.

Jamel and Markar[71] performed a meta-analysis evaluating 11 studies (n = 1906 patients) to assess both the long-term and short-term outcomes of patients managed with definitive CRT and subsequent salvage esophagectomy (n = 563) versus neoadjuvant chemoradiation followed by planned esophagectomy (n = 1343). Pooled analysis did not show any statistical difference between the groups in overall survival, postoperative mortality, pulmonary complications, and positive resection margin incidence. As alluded to previously, however, postoperative morbidity and anastomotic leak rates were statistically higher in the salvage group. A large degree of heterogeneity was present between the included studies regarding the histologic subtype of cancer (ESCC vs adenocarcinoma) and radiation dosage, with the latter contributing to the complex pathophysiology of scarring tissue planes and anastomotic leaks.[20] The investigators suggests that salvage resection be only performed in specialized multidisciplinary centers with experienced high-volume surgeons due to the complex nature and high risk for postoperative complications.[71] More importantly, patients with persistent or recurrent disease who were not fit for surgery or opted out of surgical management were not included. Therefore, the full efficacy of this treatment pathway remains unknown. Furthermore, the majority of studies included in analysis grouped both persistent and recurrent disease together for indication for salvage resection. It previously has been suggested that persistent disease may represent a more biological aggressive variant as opposed to its recurrent counterpart.[35] Further studies to distinguish between these 2 distinct patient groups still are needed considering both are eligible for salvage resection but potentially may have different prognosis.

More recently, Mitchell and colleagues[11] described their experience and perioperative outcomes among patients (n = 35) who underwent salvage esophagectomy following CRT for ESCC. Major morbidity and mortality events were observed in 71.4% (25/35) of salvage patients. No relationship was observed between radiation dose (<50.4 Gy vs ≥50.4 Gy) and incidence of major complications; 34.3% of complications in patients undergoing salvage resection were severe (Clavien-Dindo classification ≥4). Major cardiovascular events, such as arrhythmia (48.6%) and cardiac arrest (2.9%), were reported. Major pulmonary events, such as acute respiratory distress syndrome (8.6%), pneumonia (34.3%), reintubation (20%), and tracheostomy (8.6%), were seen; 30-day and 90-day mortality rates among this group were 8.6% and 17.1%, respectively. Causes of 90-day mortality included pneumonia (33%), anastomotic failure leading to tracheogastric fistula (16.6%), and respiratory failure (16.6%).[11]

Booka and colleagues[61] retrospectively examined the safety and efficacy of salvage esophagectomy after definitive CRT (fluorouracil-cisplatin regimen with total 60-Gy radiation) in patients with initially unresectable T4 ESCC: 5.7% (18/317) of nonresponders to definitive CRT underwent salvage esophagectomy; 15 of 18 (83.3%) patients underwent salvage resection for residual tumor; and 3 of 18 (16.7%) patients underwent resection for relapse. Postoperative complications included pneumonia (5.6%), anastomotic leak (38.9%), and recurrent laryngeal nerve injury (44.4%). An R0 resection was obtained in 14 of 18 patients (77.8%). Patients with upper thoracic esophageal tumors were more likely to undergo incomplete resection ($P = .011$), which was the only significant variable associated with poor overall survival on univariate Cox proportional hazards analysis ($P = .008$).[61]

As discussed previously, studies have suggested that patients with residual cancer appear to have worse survival outcomes than those with recurrence following salvage esophagectomy.[35,72] Taniyama and colleagues[73] sought to identify patients most likely to benefit from salvage resection in regard to both residual and recurrent ESCC; 100 patients were identified who failed definitive CRT (fluorouracil-cisplatin regimen with total 60-Gy radiation) and subsequently underwent salvage resection. Improved survival was observed in patients with residual cancer that had not invaded to the adventitia at the time of CRT and surgery ($P = .010$). This was not statistically significant in patients with recurrent cancer ($P = .635$). Pathologic T stage showed a correlation with survival in both the residual ($P<.001$) and recurrent ($P = .001$) patient groups. In patients with recurrent disease, improved survival was observed in those with T3 or lower disease recurrence, whereas worst survival was observed in the residual group. Nodal status before chemoradiotherapy did not confer any survival benefit in the recurrent group.

SUMMARY

Salvage resection after definitive chemotherapy for esophageal cancer is a viable treatment option for patients with persistent or recurrent disease, whether after induction or definitive CRT. Although associated with high rates of morbidity, this treatment modality offers a chance of long-term survival for patients with an otherwise grim prognosis. A selective approach can be beneficial for these patients and should be undertaken in a multidisciplinary fashion at advanced centers with high-volume and experienced surgeons. In order to optimize the outcomes in this challenging population, many factors should be considered carefully, such as the extent of radiation field, radiation dosage, choice of neoesophageal conduit, tumor location, and patients' comorbidities and underlying functional status.

CLINICS CARE POINTS

- Patients with persistent or recurrent disease after definitive CRT or induction chemoradiation with active surveillance without evidence of metastatic disease may be eligible for salvage esophagectomy

- Salvage resection should be performed in the same manner as a standard esophagectomy with special consideration toward prior radiation dosage, radiation field, and choice of conduit
- Studies have shown improved outcomes when salvage esophagectomies are performed in the setting of multidisciplinary teams and by experienced and high-volume surgeons
- Endoscopic resection may be considered for those patients with advanced locoregional disease and favorable tumor characteristics who are unfit for surgery or decline salvage resection
- When considering salvage resection and the use of a gastric conduit is prohibitory, colonic or jejunal conduits have been utilized

DISCLOSURE

The authors have no disclosures.

REFERENCES

1. Torre LA, Bray F, Siegel RL, et al. Global cancer statistics, 2012, 2012. CA Cancer J Clin 2015;65(2):87–108.
2. Esophageal Cancer — Cancer Stat Facts [Internet]. Available at: https://seer.cancer.gov/statfacts/html/esoph.html. Accessed August 21, 2020.
3. Tepper JE, Krasna M, Niedzwiecki D, et al. Phase III trial of trimodality therapy with cisplatin, fluorouracil, radiotherapy, and surgery compared with surgery alone for esophageal cancer: CALGB 9781. J Clin Oncol 2008;26(7):1086–92.
4. Sjoquist KM, Burmeister BH, Smithers BM, et al. Survival after neoadjuvant chemotherapy or chemoradiotherapy for resectable oesophageal carcinoma: An updated meta-analysis. Lancet Oncol 2011;12(7):681.
5. Van Hagen P, Hulshof MC, van Lanschot JJ, et al. Preoperative chemoradiotherapy for esophageal or junctional cancer. N Engl J Med 2012;366(22):2074.
6. Shapiro J, van Lanschot JJB, Hulshof MCCM, et al. Neoadjuvant chemoradiotherapy plus surgery versus surgery alone for oesophageal or junctional cancer (CROSS): Long-term results of a randomised controlled trial. Lancet Oncol 2015;16(9):1090.
7. Bedenne L, Michel P, Bouché O, et al. Chemoradiation followed by surgery compared with chemoradiation alone in squamous cancer of the esophagus: FFCD 9102. J Clin Oncol 2007;25(10):1160–8.
8. Teoh AY, Chiu PW, Yeung WK, et al. Long-term survival outcomes after definitive chemoradiation versus surgery in patients with resectable squamous carcinoma of the esophagus: Results from a randomized controlled trial. Ann Oncol 2013;24(1):165.
9. Stahl M, Stuschke M, Lehmann N, et al. Chemoradiation with and without surgery in patients with locally advanced squamous cell carcinoma of the esophagus. J Clin Oncol 2005;23(10):2310.
10. Farinella E, Safar A, Nasser HA, et al. Salvage esophagectomy after failure of definitive radiochemotherapy for esophageal cancer. J Surg Oncol 2016;114(7):833.
11. Mitchell KG, Nelson DB, Corsini EM, et al. Morbidity following salvage esophagectomy for squamous cell carcinoma: The MD Anderson experience. Dis Esophagus 2020;33(3):doz067.

12. Hoeben A, Polak J, Van De Voorde L, et al. Cervical esophageal cancer: A gap in cancer knowledge. Ann Oncol 2016;27(9):1664.

13. Cooper JS, Guo MD, Herskovic A, et al. Chemoradiotherapy of locally advanced esophageal cancer: long-term follow-up of a prospective randomized trial (RTOG 85-01). Radiation Therapy Oncology Group. JAMA 1999;281(17):1623.

14. Minsky BD, Pajak TF, Ginsberg RJ, et al. INT 0123 (Radiation therapy oncology group 94-05) phase III trial of combined-modality therapy for esophageal cancer: High-dose versus standard-dose radiation therapy. J Clin Oncol 2002;20(5): 1167.

15. Van Der Wilk BJ, Eyck BM, Spaander MCW, et al. Towards an organ-sparing approach for locally advanced esophageal cancer. Dig Surg 2019;36(6):462–9.

16. Swisher SG, Wynn P, Putnam JB, et al. Salvage esophagectomy for recurrent tumors after definitive chemotherapy and radiotherapy. J Thorac Cardiovasc Surg 2002;123(1):175.

17. Nakamura T, Hayashi K, Ota M, et al. Salvage esophagectomy after definitive chemotherapy and radiotherapy for advanced esophageal cancer. Am J Surg 2004;188(3):261.

18. Tomimaru Y, Yano M, Takachi K, et al. Factors affecting the prognosis of patients with esophageal cancer undergoing salvage surgery after definitive chemoradiotherapy. J Surg Oncol 2006;93(5):422.

19. Chao YK, Chan SC, Chang HK, et al. Salvage surgery after failed chemoradiotherapy in squamous cell carcinoma of the esophagus. Eur J Surg Oncol 2009; 35(3):289.

20. Oki E, Morita M, Kakeji Y, et al. Salvage esophagectomy after definitive chemoradiotherapy for esophageal cancer. Dis Esophagus 2007;20(4):301.

21. Borghesi S, Hawkins MA, Tait D. Oesophagectomy after definitive chemoradiation in patients with locally advanced oesophageal cancer. Clin Oncol 2008; 20(3):221–6.

22. Nishimura M, Daiko H, Yoshida J, et al. Salvage esophagectomy following definitive chemoradiotherapy. Gen Thorac Cardiovasc Surg 2007;55(11):461.

23. Marks JL, Hofstetter W, Correa AM, et al. Salvage esophagectomy after failed definitive chemoradiation for esophageal adenocarcinoma. Ann Thorac Surg 2012;94(4):1126.

24. Tachimori Y, Kanamori N, Uemura N, et al. Salvage esophagectomy after high-dose chemoradiotherapy for esophageal squamous cell carcinoma. J Thorac Cardiovasc Surg 2009;137(1):49–54.

25. Ishikura S, Nihei K, Ohtsu A, et al. Long-term toxicity after definitive chemoradiotherapy for squamous cell carcinoma of the thoracic esophagus. J Clin Oncol 2003;21(14):2697.

26. Hironaka S, Ohtsu A, Boku N, et al. Nonrandomized comparison between definitive chemoradiotherapy and radical surgery in patients with T2-3Nany M0 squamous cell carcinoma of the esophagus. Int J Radiat Oncol Biol Phys 2003;57(2): 425–33.

27. Meunier B, Raoul J, Le Prisé E, et al. Salvage esophagectomy after unsuccessful curative chemoradiotherapy for squamous cell cancer of the esophagus. Dig Surg 1998;15(3):224.

28. Murakami M, Kuroda Y, Okamoto Y, et al. Neoadjuvant concurrent chemoradiotherapy followed by definitive high-dose radiotherapy or surgery for operable thoracic esophageal carcinoma. Int J Radiat Oncol Biol Phys 1998;40(5):1049.

29. Cunningham D, Allum WH, Stenning SP, et al. Perioperative chemotherapy versus surgery alone for resectable gastroesophageal cancer. N Engl J Med 2006; 355(1):11.

30. Taketa T, Xiao L, Sudo K, et al. Propensity-based matching between esophago-gastric cancer patients who had surgery and who declined surgery after preoperative chemoradiation. Oncology 2013;85(2):95.

31. Castoro C, Scarpa M, Cagol M, et al. Complete clinical response after neoadjuvant chemoradiotherapy for squamous cell cancer of the thoracic oesophagus: is surgery always necessary? J Gastrointest Surg 2013;17(8):1375–81.

32. Haefner MF, Lang K, Verma V, et al. Neoadjuvant versus definitive chemoradiotherapy for locally advanced esophageal cancer: Outcomes and patterns of failure. Strahlentherapie Onkol 2018;194(2):116–24.

33. Franko J, Voynov G, Goldman CD. Esophagectomy timing after neoadjuvant therapy for distal esophageal adenocarcinoma. Ann Thorac Surg 2016;101(3):1123.

34. Gardner-Thorpe J, Hardwick RH, Dwerryhouse SJ. Salvage oesophagectomy after local failure of definitive chemoradiotherapy. Br J Surg 2007;94(9):1059.

35. Markar S, Gronnier C, Duhamel A, et al. Salvage surgery after chemoradiotherapy in the management of esophageal cancer: Is it a viable therapeutic option? J Clin Oncol 2015;33(33):3866–73.

36. Kim JY, Correa AM, Vaporciyan AA, et al. Does the timing of esophagectomy after chemoradiation affect outcome? Ann Thorac Surg 2012;93(1):207.

37. Levinsky NC, Wima K, Morris MC, et al. Outcome of delayed versus timely esophagectomy after chemoradiation for esophageal adenocarcinoma. J Thorac Cardiovasc Surg 2020;159(6):2555–66.

38. Keller SM, Ryan LM, Coia LR, et al. High dose chemoradiotherapy followed by esophagectomy for adenocarcinoma of the esophagus and gastroesophageal junction: Results of a phase II study of the eastern cooperative oncology group. Cancer 1998;83(9):1908–16.

39. Blencowe NS, Strong S, McNair AG, et al. Reporting of short-term clinical outcomes after esophagectomy: A systematic review. Ann Surg 2012;255(4):658.

40. Wormuth JK, Heitmiller RF. Esophageal Conduit Necrosis. Thorac Surg Clin 2006; 16(1):11.

41. Athanasiou A, Hennessy M, Spartalis E, et al. Conduit necrosis following esophagectomy: An up-to-date literature review. World J Gastrointest Surg 2019;11(3): 155–68.

42. Bludau M, Vallböhmer D, Gutschow C, et al. Quantitative measurement of gastric mucosal microcirculation using a combined laser Doppler flowmeter and spectrophotometer. Dis Esophagus 2008;21(7):668.

43. Karliczek A, Benaron DA, Baas PC, et al. Intraoperative assessment of microperfusion with visible light spectroscopy in esophageal and colorectal anastomoses. Eur Surg Res 2008;41(3):303.

44. Pacheco PE, Hill SM, Henriques SM, et al. The novel use of intraoperative laser-induced fluorescence of indocyanine green tissue angiography for evaluation of the gastric conduit in esophageal reconstructive surgery. Am J Surg 2013; 205(3):349.

45. Kitagawa H, Namikawa T, Iwabu J, et al. Assessment of the blood supply using the indocyanine green fluorescence method and postoperative endoscopic evaluation of anastomosis of the gastric tube during esophagectomy. Surg Endosc 2018;32(4):1749–54.

46. Koyanagi K, Ozawa S, Oguma J, et al. Blood flow speed of the gastric conduit assessed by indocyanine green fluorescence: New predictive evaluation of anastomotic leakage after esophagectomy. Med (United States) 2016;95(30):e4386.

47. Kumagai Y, Ishiguro T, Haga N, et al. Hemodynamics of the reconstructed gastric tube during esophagectomy: Assessment of outcomes with indocyanine green fluorescence. World J Surg 2014;38(1):138.

48. Murawa D, Hünerbein M, Spychała A, et al. Indocyanine green angiography for evaluation of gastric conduit perfusion during esophagectomy - First experience. Acta Clin Belg 2012;112(4):275–80.

49. Ohi M, Toiyama Y, Mohri Y, et al. Prevalence of anastomotic leak and the impact of indocyanine green fluorescein imaging for evaluating blood flow in the gastric conduit following esophageal cancer surgery. Esophagus 2017;14(4):351.

50. Rino Y, Yukawa N, Sato T, et al. Visualization of blood supply route to the reconstructed stomach by indocyanine green fluorescence imaging during esophagectomy. BMC Med Imaging 2014;14:18.

51. Sarkaria IS, Bains MS, Finley DJ, et al. Intraoperative near-infrared fluorescence imaging as an adjunct to robotic-assisted minimally invasive esophagectomy. Innov Technol Tech Cardiothorac Vasc Surg 2014;9(5):391–3.

52. Shimada Y, Okumura T, Nagata T, et al. Usefulness of blood supply visualization by indocyanine green fluorescence for reconstruction during esophagectomy. Esophagus 2011;8(4):259–66.

53. Yukaya T, Saeki H, Kasagi Y, et al. Indocyanine Green Fluorescence Angiography for Quantitative Evaluation of Gastric Tube Perfusion in Patients Undergoing Esophagectomy. J Am Coll Surg 2015;221(2):e37.

54. Zehetner J, DeMeester SR, Alicuben ET, et al. Intraoperative assessment of perfusion of the gastric graft and correlation with anastomotic leaks after esophagectomy. Ann Surg 2015;262(1):74.

55. Athanasiou A, Spartalis E, Spartalis M, et al. Management of oesophageal perforation based on the Pittsburgh Perforation Severity Score: Still a matter of debate. Eur J Cardio-thoracic Surg 2020;57(1):198.

56. Scott-Wittenborn N, Jackson RS. Intraoperative imaging during minimally invasive transoral robotic surgery using near-infrared light. Am J Otolaryngol Head Neck Med Surg 2018;39(2):220–2.

57. Ladak F, Dang JT, Switzer N, et al. Indocyanine green for the prevention of anastomotic leaks following esophagectomy: a meta-analysis. Surg Endosc 2019; 33(2):384–94.

58. Juloori A, Tucker SL, Komaki R, et al. Influence of preoperative radiation field on postoperative leak rates in esophageal cancer patients after trimodality therapy. J Thorac Oncol 2014;9(4):534.

59. Hofstetter WL. Salvage esophagectomy. J Thorac Dis 2014;6(Suppl 3):S341.

60. Sepesi B, Swisher SG, Walsh GL, et al. Omental reinforcement of the thoracic esophagogastric anastomosis: an analysis of leak and reintervention rates in patients undergoing planned and salvage esophagectomy. J Thorac Cardiovasc Surg 2012;144(5):1146.

61. Booka E, Haneda R, Ishii K, et al. Appropriate Candidates for Salvage Esophagectomy of Initially Unresectable Locally Advanced T4 Esophageal Squamous Cell Carcinoma. Ann Surg Oncol 2020;27(9):3163–70.

62. Oezcelik A, Banki F, DeMeester SR, et al. Delayed esophagogastrostomy: a safe strategy for management of patients with ischemic gastric conduit at time of esophagectomy. J Am Coll Surg 2009;208(6):1030–4.

63. Swisher SG, DeFord L, Merriman KW, et al. Effect of operative volume on morbidity, mortality, and hospital use after esophagectomy for cancer. J Thorac Cardiovasc Surg 2000;119(6):1126.

64. Fujita H, Yamana H, Sueyoshi S, et al. Impact on outcome of additional microvascular anastomosis-supercharge- on colon interposition for esophageal replacement: Comparative and multivariate analysis. World J Surg 1997;21(9):998–1003.

65. Kesler KA, Pillai ST, Birdas TJ, et al. "Supercharged" isoperistaltic colon interposition for long-segment esophageal reconstruction. Ann Thorac Surg 2013;95(4): 1162.

66. Swisher SG, Hofstetter WL, Miller MJ. The supercharged microvascular jejunal interposition. Semin Thorac Cardiovasc Surg 2007;19(1):56–65.

67. Baker CR, Forshaw MJ, Gossage JA, et al. Long-term outcome and quality of life after supercharged jejunal interposition for oesophageal replacement. Surgeon 2015;13(4):187.

68. Ascioti AJ, Hofstetter WL, Miller MJ, et al. Long-segment, supercharged, pedicled jejunal flap for total esophageal reconstruction. J Thorac Cardiovasc Surg 2005;130(5):1391.

69. Makazu M, Kato K, Takisawa H, et al. Feasibility of endoscopic mucosal resection as salvage treatment for patients with local failure after definitive chemoradiotherapy for stage IB, II, and III esophageal squamous cell cancer. Dis Esophagus 2014;27(1):42.

70. Kanamori J, Abe S, Kurita D, et al. Minimally invasive hybrid surgery: A salvage tumor enucleation for local recurrence of thoracic esophageal carcinoma after definitive chemoradiotherapy. Asian J Endosc Surg 2020;14(1):77–80.

71. Jamel S, Markar SR. Salvage esophagectomy: Safe therapeutic strategy? J Thorac Dis 2017;9(Suppl 8):S799.

72. Watanabe M, Mine S, Nishida K, et al. Salvage esophagectomy after definitive chemoradiotherapy for patients with esophageal squamous cell carcinoma: who really benefits from this high-risk surgery? Ann Surg Oncol 2015;22(13): 4438.

73. Taniyama Y, Sakurai T, Heishi T, et al. Different strategy of salvage esophagectomy between residual and recurrent esophageal cancer after definitive chemoradiotherapy. J Thorac Dis 2018;10(3):1554–62.

74. Bakshi A, Sugarbaker DJ, Burt BM. Alternative conduits for esophageal replacement. Ann Cardiothorac Surg 2017;6(2):137.

75. Sugarbaker D, Bueno R, Burt BM, et al. Sugarbaker's Adult chest surgery. 3rd edition. New York: McGraw-Hill Education/Medical; 2020.

76. Yasuda T, Shiozaki H. Esophageal reconstruction with colon tissue. Surg Today 2011;41(6):745.

77. DeMeester SR. Colonic interposition for benign disease. Oper Tech Thorac Cardiovasc Surg 2006;11(3):232–49.

78. Strauss DC, Forshaw MJ, Tandon RC, et al. Surgical management of colonic redundancy following esophageal replacement. Dis Esophagus 2008;21(3):E1.

79. Saeki H, Morita M, Harada N, et al. Esophageal replacement by colon interposition with microvascular surgery for patients with thoracic esophageal cancer: The utility of superdrainage. Dis Esophagus 2013;26(1):50.

Consolidation Therapy in Esophageal Cancer

Jeremiah T. Martin, MBBCh, MSCRD, FRCSI

KEYWORDS

- Consolidation therapy • Esophageal cancer treatment • Adjuvant therapy
- Multimodality therapy

KEY POINTS

- For surgical patients, consider tumor response, margin status, and numbers of lymph nodes examined and proportion positive.
- For nonsurgical patients, consider performance status, tumor biomarkers, and regimen used to this point in therapy.
- Multidisciplinary discussion and monitoring of the plan of care is critical in selecting patients for consolidation therapy.

The overall goal of cancer therapy is to reduce the tumor cell population to zero.[1] In the case of esophageal cancer, this is accomplished most frequently using multimodality therapy, where chemotherapy, radiation, and surgery, are used to affect the best oncologic outcome.[2–7] The term consolidation is generally used to describe dose intensification strategies or additional treatment performed following completion of the primary regimen. The objective is to reduce locoregional and distant recurrence and improve progression-free and overall survival. Consolidation is a common strategy in hematologic malignancies and is increasingly explored in other cancer types including breast[8] and lung[9] when appropriate.

The role of consolidation in esophageal cancer falls into 2 broad categories:

- Patients who have completed multimodality therapy, including surgery, and are found to have risk factors on final pathology that might benefit from additional adjuvant therapy
- Patients who have completed neoadjuvant therapy but for any reason do not proceed to surgery, or patients who have received definitive chemoradiation (dCRT) but demonstrate persistent disease on restaging

Esophageal cancer is a systemic problem. Although screening continues to improve, most patients still present with advanced-stage disease. A recent review of SEER

Thoracic Surgery, Southern Ohio Medical Center, 1711 27th Street, Braunlin Building, Suite 206, Portsmouth, OH 45662, USA
E-mail address: martinjt@somc.org

Surg Clin N Am 101 (2021) 483–488
https://doi.org/10.1016/j.suc.2021.03.009
0039-6109/21/© 2021 Elsevier Inc. All rights reserved.

surgical.theclinics.com

(Surveillance, Epidemiology, and End Results Program) data demonstrated that at this time less than 20% of patients present with stage I cancer.[10] Therefore, most patients will require chemotherapy and radiation with or without surgery. Over the past several decades, multiple studies have been conducted to understand the optimal sequencing of, and appropriate combinations of, chemotherapy and radiation in conjunction with surgery. In the United States, it is now generally accepted that preoperative chemoradiation followed by surgery in appropriate patients will ensure the best outcomes.[4,11] Another recent review of the SEER and NCDB (National Cancer Database) databases demonstrates that although there are variations in the types of operations that are chosen for esophageal and esophagogastric cancers, the factors that most strongly predict long-term survival are tumor biology and completeness of multimodality therapy.[7] Tumor histology (adenocarcinoma vs squamous cell) is closely linked with prognosis and as such drives different staging algorithms and guides treatment.[4]

ROLE OF ADJUVANT CHEMOTHERAPY AFTER SURGERY

Although many patients are treated with trimodality therapy, clinical stage T1 and T2 patients are appropriately offered surgical resection as definitive therapy. For some, the operation itself can be curative. Although less frequently discussed, a role for adjuvant chemotherapy has been well established in these early stage patients. A second group is comprised of patients clinically staged as T1 and T2 who pathologically are found to have positive lymph nodes.

In 2003, Ando and colleagues[12] published their phase 3 trial to compare survival with surgery alone and to surgery and postoperative adjuvant chemotherapy with 2 courses of cisplatin and fluorouracil (FP) in patients with resected esophageal squamous cell carcinoma. This study concluded that there was a significant 5-year disease-free survival (DFS) benefit from postoperative adjuvant chemotherapy with FP in the group of patients with positive lymph nodes. This study has subsequently been supported by others.[13]

THE ROLE OF CONSOLIDATION AFTER SURGERY

If one accepts that adjuvant chemotherapy for node-positive R0 resection patients is beneficial, can one make the same assumption following completion of trimodality therapy? Data following trimodality therapy demonstrate that patients are at higher risk for recurrence and death if they have positive nodes and that risk increases further with more positive nodes. In chemotherapy-naive patients, there are data to support chemotherapy,[12,13] but do those data extend to patients who have already received trimodality therapy?

It is accepted that patients with complete response at time of surgery have better survival than those with residual viable tumor; those patients in turn have better survival than those with residual active lymph node involvement. Frequently the assumption is that those who are more likely to recur are the ones most likely to benefit. In the case of esophageal cancer and consolidation therapy, this remains unclear.

Following a successful resection, the pathologist report provides gold standard information on tumor biology and on response to chemotherapy and radiation. Margin status, lymph node status, and degree of response are important prognostic factors and may be used to select which patients may benefit from consolidation therapy.[4]

Important considerations include:

- Tumor response (tumor regression is graded from complete response through near complete, partial, and poor or no response)

- Numbers of lymph nodes examined and proportion positive
- Margin status: complete resection (R0), microscopic positive margin (R1), and macroscopic or gross residual disease (R2).

By current guidelines for squamous cell carcinoma, in the absence of gross residual disease, no additional therapy is warranted assuming the patient has tolerated a complete course of neoadjuvant therapy if such was required.[4] For adenocarcinoma, lymph node positivity or significant residual tumor should prompt a discussion of the potential benefits of adjuvant therapy. It should be noted that there is no strong evidence available at this point that can be applied to all patients. This article will review some of the available data and discuss some potential future directions.

Sun and colleagues[14] evaluated the clinical efficacy of consolidation chemotherapy in resectable esophageal squamous cell carcinoma after trimodality therapy. Over a 7-year period, 192 patients were enrolled. Of these, 72 underwent consolidation chemotherapy. For these patients, an additional 1 to 4 cycles of chemotherapy similar to their preoperative regimen (cisplatin, fluorouracil) were administered. Five-year survival was not different between the 2 groups; however, the progression-free survival was slightly better at 38% in the consolidation group, compared with 34% in the standard group. Multivariable modeling demonstrated that progression-free survival was most notably worse in males and those who did not achieve a pathologic complete response.

For many clinicians, the presence of persistently positive lymph nodes after resection will generally prompt a discussion about potential benefits of adjuvant chemotherapy. After all, the purpose of the resection following CRT is to remove residual viable disease, so arguments for and against are reasonable. As stated, there is not strong evidence to help predict which patients may benefit from additional therapy.

The particular case of adenocarcinoma and consolidation therapy following trimodality treatment is the topic of a recently reported study by Bott and colleagues[15] from the United Kingdom. Six hundred sixteen patients were included in this analysis (243 of these had microscopically positive margins and were excluded from analysis). Poor survival was predicted by pN status, poor differentiation, and poor treatment response. The benefit of adjuvant chemotherapy did not reach independent significance compared with no additional treatment after resection. A slightly longer survival was observed in patients undergoing consolidation therapy who had demonstrated a good treatment response, but this too did not reach statistical significance (hazard ratio [HR] 0.65, 95% confidence interval [CI] 0.4–1.06, $P=.087$)

Li and colleagues report a novel approach[16,17] to not only evaluating the binary condition of whether lymph nodes are positive, but also take into consideration the relationship of adequacy of lymph node dissection to this outcome. Their study enrolled 298 patients with squamous cell carcinoma who underwent esophagectomy. Adjuvant therapy included standard of care therapy directed by current standard guidelines. A multivariable model was constructed including total number of resected lymph nodes, lymph node positive ratio, and lymph node stage. In contrast to using each of these as single factors, the combination of total lymph nodes resected and lymph node ratio was found to be highly predictive of the value of adjuvant therapy in this cohort. A strategy such as this may be useful in future studies in esophageal adenocarcinoma and in the overall benefit of consolidation therapy in general.

CONSOLIDATION IN THE NONSURGICAL PATIENT

There is a role for consolidation therapy in patients who initially were considered for trimodality therapy, but later because of patient preference, loss of performance status during neoadjuvant therapy, or progression of comorbidities may be ineligible for surgery. Fang and colleagues[18] evaluated this specific patient cohort and published their findings. Over a 12-year period, 190 patients failed to proceed to surgery after neoadjuvant chemoradiation. Evaluation focused on patterns of recurrence, and in particular outcomes in those patients who had a clinical complete response. All patients underwent consolidation chemoradiation, which in this series involved 1 additional round of chemoradiation to extend the neoadjuvant protocol. Interestingly, the overall 5-year survival was 40%, with cancer recurrence being identified in 60% of the patients who had clinical complete response, and local recurrence was the most common failure pattern. Endoscopic findings during surveillance were of highest predictive value. Notably, patients with normal endoscopy after completing therapy have the lowest rate of local recurrence.

The effects of consolidation chemotherapy following dCRT in patients with esophageal squamous cell cancer was reported by Wu and colleagues.[19] Over a 3-year period, the outcomes of 522 patients undergoing dCRT were evaluated. Two hundred nine patients achieved clinical complete response, and of these, 67 received consolidation therapy. Thirty-four patients received an additional 2 cycles of the same 5-FU and cisplatin regimen used initially, while 33 received 2 cycles of docetaxel with cisplatin or nedaplatin. Consolidation did not prolong progression-free survival; however, it did improve median overall survival from 27 to 53 months. This study with robust propensity matching concluded that consolidation therapy did not improve progression-free survival, but may offer extended overall survival in those patients who achieve complete clinical response after dCRT.

Despite these promising results, other studies report conflicting analyses. In 2017, the outcomes of 812 patients with stage 2 to 3 esophageal squamous cell carcinoma, treated with dCRT, were reported.[20] Propensity matching was used to create study groups whose patients underwent consolidation versus observation after dCRT. In this study, there were no significant differences in local or regional failure and no differences in overall survival for these patients with stage 2 to 3 squamous cell carcinoma of the esophagus.

FUTURE DIRECTIONS

Esophageal cancer in particular presents several novel options, which, although not part of frontline therapy at this time, are opportunity for further clinical trials development that may lead to advances in the arena of consolidation therapy.

In 2017 in the Pacific Trial, patients with stage 3 lung cancer who underwent dCRT were treated with consolidation therapy using durvalumab.[9] The treatment resulted in significant increases in disease-free survival, progression-free survival, and median time to death of 28.3 months in the durvalumab arm versus 16.2 months in the placebo arm. Duralumab is a highly selective human immunoglobulin g 1 (IgG1) monoclonal antibody that blocks PD-L1 bingeing to PD-1 and CD80, allowing T cells to recognize and kill tumor cells. It is theorized that chemoradiotherapy may up-regulate PD-L1 expression in tumor cells.

A recent publication from the Cochrane database suggested benefit from additional targeted agents.[21] In the setting of palliative therapy, an overall survival in favor of the group receiving palliative chemotherapy and/or targeted therapy compared with best supportive care (HR 0.81, 95% CI 0.71–0.92, high-quality evidence) was reported. Ramucirumab was found to improve both overall survival and progression-free survival in this patient population. Moving forward, applications of targeted therapies in patients completing therapy are likely to be investigated further.

Current guidelines suggest that in patients with locally advanced, recurrent, or metastatic tumors, additional testing of pathology specimens should be undertaken. HER2 expression may be evaluated, and next-generation sequencing allows for evaluation of numerous simultaneous mutations. Microsatellite instability and mismatch repair in addition to PDL1 testing may also allow patients to be treated with novel PD-1 inhibitors.[4] Although these biomarker tests are not routine for frontline therapy at this time, in any conversation about consolidation therapy, they should be considered by the multidisciplinary tumor board discussing challenging cases.

SUMMARY

Review of available studies and data at this time indicates that the optimal treatment of esophageal cancer is multimodality therapy. The data to support routine use of consolidation therapy are weak at this time. Nevertheless, in specific cases, an argument for additional treatment can be made, guided by multidisciplinary discussion. Consolidation should strongly be considered in patients who have completed all courses of therapy including surgery yet have significant numbers of positive lymph nodes, poor tumor response, or microscopic/macroscopic positive margins after resection. Where possible, opportunity to enroll such patients in clinical trials should be sought such that additional information may be gained to guide future treatment pathways. In the coming years, it is likely that studies will demonstrate benefit to routine biomarker testing and consideration of novel therapeutic agents to optimize survival.

CLINICS CARE POINTS

- In a patient who has received surgical therapy, the need for adjuvant therapy should be discussed at a multidisciplinary conference.
- Consolidation therapy should be considered in patients who may no longer be surgical candidates after neoadjuvant therapy.
- The goals of consolidation therapy are to maximize tumor control after primary treatment; therefore delays should be avoided if possible.
- The field of medical oncology continues to rapidly evolve; in each clinical case, available targeted agents should be considered as new options become available.

REFERENCES

1. Jasmin Jo PW. Principles of chemotherapy. In: Youmans J, editor. Youmans neurological surgery. Philadelphia (PA): Saunders/Elsevier; 2011. p. 923-7.
2. Cunningham D, Allum WH, Stenning SP, et al. Perioperative chemotherapy versus surgery alone for resectable gastroesophageal cancer. N Engl J Med 2006; 355(1):11-20.
3. Macdonald JS, Smalley SR, Benedetti J, et al. Chemoradiotherapy after surgery compared with surgery alone for adenocarcinoma of the stomach or gastro-esophageal junction. N Engl J Med 2001;345(10):725-30.
4. National Comprehensive Cancer N. Esophageal and esophagogastric junction cancers (version 1.2020). Available at: https://www.nccn.org/professionals/physician_gls/pdf/esophageal.pdf.
5. Stahl M, Walz MK, Stuschke M, et al. Phase III comparison of preoperative chemotherapy compared with chemoradiotherapy in patients with locally

advanced adenocarcinoma of the esophagogastric junction. J Clin Oncol 2009; 27(6):851–6.

6. van Hagen P, Hulshof MCCM, van Lanschot JJB, et al. Preoperative chemoradio-therapy for esophageal or junctional cancer. N Engl J Med 2012;366(22): 2074–84.

7. Martin JT, Mahan A, Zwischenberger JB, et al. Should gastric cardia cancers be treated with esophagectomy or total gastrectomy? A comprehensive analysis of 4,996 NSQIP/SEER patients. J Am Coll Surg 2015;220(4):510–20.

8. Hurvitz SA. Dose intensification of chemotherapy for early breast cancer in the age of de-escalation. Lancet 2019;393(10179):1390–2.

9. Antonia SJ, Villegas A, Daniel D, et al. Durvalumab after chemoradiotherapy in stage III non-small-cell lung cancer. N Engl J Med 2017;377(20):1919–29.

10. Zeng Y, Ruan W, Liu J, et al. Esophageal cancer in patients under 50: a SEER analysis. J Thorac Dis 2018;10(5):2542–50.

11. Shahbaz Sarwar CM, Luketich JD, Landreneau RJ, et al. Esophageal cancer: an update. Int J Surg 2010;8(6):417–22.

12. Ando N, Iizuka T, Ide H, et al. Surgery plus chemotherapy compared with surgery alone for localized squamous cell carcinoma of the thoracic esophagus: a Japan Clinical Oncology Group Study–JCOG9204. J Clin Oncol 2003;21(24):4592–6.

13. Lee J, Lee KE, Im YH, et al. Adjuvant chemotherapy with 5-fluorouracil and cisplatin in lymph node-positive thoracic esophageal squamous cell carcinoma. Ann Thorac Surg 2005;80(4):1170–5.

14. Sun Y, Cheng S, Lu Y, et al. The clinical efficacy of consolidation chemotherapy for resectable esophageal squamous cell cancer after trimodality therapy. J Cancer Res Ther 2016;12(1):90–5.

15. Bott R, Zylstra J, Wilkinson M, et al. P96 the current role of adjuvant therapy in patients following neo-adjuvant chemotherapy and r0 resection for lower oeso-phageal and goj adenocarcinoma. Dis Esophagus 2019;32(Supplement_2).

16. McCloskey D, Shersher DD. Does a lymph node-based model predict clinical value for adjuvant therapy in squamous cell carcinoma of the esophagus treated with upfront surgery? Ann Surg Oncol 2019;26(8):2313–5.

17. Li Y, Zhao W, Ni J, et al. Predicting the value of adjuvant therapy in esophageal squamous cell carcinoma by combining the total number of examined lymph no-des with the positive lymph. Ann Surg 2019;26(8):2367–74.

18. Fang H-Y, Chao Y-K, Chang H-K, et al. Survival outcomes of consolidation che-moradiotherapy in esophageal cancer patients who achieve clinical complete response but refuse surgery after neoadjuvant chemoradiotherapy. Dis Esoph-agus 2017;30(2):1–8.

19. Wu S-X, Li X-Y, Xu H-Y, et al. Effect of consolidation chemotherapy following definitive chemoradiotherapy in patients with esophageal squamous cell cancer. Sci Rep 2017;7(1):16870.

20. Chen Y, Guo L, Cheng X, et al. With or without consolidation chemotherapy using cisplatin/5-FU after concurrent chemoradiotherapy in stage II–III squamous cell carcinoma of the esophagus: a propensity score-matched analysis. Radiother Oncol 2018;129(1):154–60.

21. Janmaat VT, Steyerberg EW, van der Gaast A, et al. Palliative chemotherapy and targeted therapies for esophageal and gastroesophageal junction cancer. Co-chrane Database Syst Rev 2017;11:CD004063.

Surgeons' Role in Local Palliation of Esophageal Cancer

John A. Federico, MD, FRCSC[a],*,
Jeremiah T. Martin, MBBCh, MSCRD, FRCSI[b]

KEYWORDS

- Palliation • Esophageal cancer treatment • Adjuvant therapy • Multimodality therapy

KEY POINTS

- Esophageal cancer commonly presents in advanced stage, and many patients can benefit from palliative intervention.
- Palliation includes management of digestive obstruction, tracheal esophageal fistulas, malnutrition, and pain. Endoscopic stenting remains an excellent first-line therapy; however, this should be discussed in a multidisciplinary setting, taking into account expectations for long-term survival and the risk of complications, which are time dependent, as a stent remains in place for longer periods.
- Advanced endoscopic skills and an understanding of the technical approaches to palliation as well as an understanding of how these patients can benefit are essential to achieve success.

PALLIATION OF ESOPHAGEAL CANCER

Esophageal cancer is the eighth most common cancer worldwide, and the sixth most common cause of cancer-related death.[1] In the United States, the proportion of patients with esophageal cancer found to have adenocarcinoma has increased. Overall, the median and 5-year survival remains poor (10 months and 22%) with most of the patients continuing to present with advanced stage disease.[2] It is not surprising, therefore, that many patients will require palliative interventions to improve quality of life.

Palliative care is defined as medical care focused on the relief of suffering and support for the best possible quality of life for patients facing serious life-threatening illness.[3] For patients with esophageal cancer, it is common for patients to develop symptoms and complications related to their primary esophageal cancer site as

[a] Kalispell Regional Healthcare, 1333 Surgical Services Drive, Kalispell, MT 59901, USA;
[b] Southern Ohio Medical Center, 1711 27th Street, Braunlin Building, Suite 206, Portsmouth, OH 45662, USA
* Corresponding author.
E-mail address: jfederico@krmc.org

Surg Clin N Am 101 (2021) 489–497
https://doi.org/10.1016/j.suc.2021.03.010
0039-6109/21/© 2021 Elsevier Inc. All rights reserved.

surgical.theclinics.com

well as metastatic disease. Local disease frequently leads to dysphagia, obstruction, bleeding, nutritional issues, and pain.[4] Distant disease may include bone pain, pleural effusion, and ascites.

In addition to chemotherapy and radiation therapy (CRT), the following local therapies have been investigated, and all may play a role in improving the quality of life of patients with advanced esophageal cancer[4–6]:

- Endoscopic dilatation
- Endoscopic stenting
- Surgical resection
- Brachytherapy
- Photodynamic therapy
- Endoscopic laser therapy
- Endoscopic chemotherapy
- Argon plasma coagulation
- Cryotherapy
- Feeding tube placement in conjunction with dilatation and/or stenting
- Surgical bypass

Initial Evaluation and Assessment

Each patient should be evaluated by a team familiar with the disease and its treatments but also with complications that occur as a result of the disease. Experience allows this team to assess the individual patient's needs and their ability to tolerate treatment by optimizing palliation. Standardized tools exist to help the health care team, including the Karnofsky and the Eastern Cooperative Oncology Group (ECOG) performance scores and the dysphagia grading system.[4] The team should be led by a physician who has ample experience and directs the patient care to be provided. Ideally this consists of a surgeon/endoscopist, radiation oncologist, palliative care clinician, nutritionist, and care coordinator. The various local therapy options are explored; however, as a general principle, expected survival in addition to ability to withstand purposed treatment should be considered. Importantly, although endoscopic stenting provides immediate symptomatic improvement in terms of secretion management and ability to swallow, the complications of stents and lesser durability compared with radiation or chemoradiation should be considered.[6–8]

Esophageal Obstruction

Tumors causing obstruction of the esophagus are common. Patients frequently present with months of slight dysphagia, which then rapidly progresses to profound dysphagia, weight loss, and malnutrition. Frequently, this prompts aggressive work-up for staging and appointments for evaluation. While awaiting these steps the symptoms can progress quickly. In such cases dilation, stenting, and feeding tubes can all be considered. Coordinating and making the right choices can be a challenge. Often patients facing a new diagnosis are reluctant to agree to feeding tubes due to a lack of understanding and the benefit. In our practice we spend time explaining the benefits nutrition and hydration provides. Allowing simple hydration enables patients to remain in the comfort of their home and equally as importantly maintain their treatment regimen without interruption due to hospitalization or emergency room visits.

Endoscopic Dilatation and Stenting

For the esophageal surgeon, having endoscopic skillsets is paramount to being able to provide palliative therapies for these patients. The endoscopist needs to assess the location of the lesion, the length of the lesion, and the degree of obstruction. Biopsies are performed to establish cell type and biological behavior of malignancy. Endoscopic dilatation can then be performed with balloon dilator or bougie over guidewire with the objective of establishing a lumen adequate enough to allow for the passage of liquids (**Fig. 1**). Generally, this will be a caliber of approximately 11 or 12 mm. For soft foods, a caliber of 14 to 15 mm needs to be achieved. The objective early on is to reestablish esophageal continuity for the passage of nourishing liquids and to alleviate the aspiration of saliva. If palliative CRT is then pursued, a more normal oral diet may then be reestablished after several weeks of treatment.

Repetitive endoscopic dilatation procedures can provide some measure of relief of dysphagia, but generally symptoms will return within 7 to 10 days if no other options are pursued. Of course, repetitive dilatations run the ever-present risk of perforation before or during CRT, which might necessitate the pursuit of surgical resection as an option for palliation or more likely the deployment of an endoluminal stent to prevent sepsis of the patient and in effect, accelerate their demise. It is with these issues to consider that necessitates this endoscopic skillset in the hands of the surgeon or at the very least, a cooperative and collaborative relationship with a gastroenterologist so that in the event of a perforation, resection or stenting can be accomplished in short order.

Self-expanding metal stents (SEMS) came into existence in the mid-1990s and offer an attractive approach in the palliation of esophageal cancer. Stenting will offer immediate improvement in dysphagia and secretion management; however, long-term indwelling stents are known to have complications. Stents are available both in covered and uncovered varieties, with the primary advantage of covered stents being the limitation of tumor ingrowth.[4]

SEMS in an obstructed patient will achieve the palliative goal of management of saliva, prevention of aspiration, relief of fatigue and coughing, and allow one to address hydration and nutrition.

Stents come in various lengths and diameters as well as being fully covered or partially covered (**Fig. 2**). A partially covered stent migrates less and should be selected for patients with a predicted shorter lifespan. A fully covered stent has less propensity for tissue overgrowth at either end and is easier to remove at a later date if the patient is to have therapeutic CRT. These stents are more prone to migration, but the tendency can be mitigated by proper size (width) selection and the placement of proximal clips at the mouth of the stent. After initial deployment of a stent, a balloon dilator can be used to "fix" the stent in position and assist with the proximal or distal

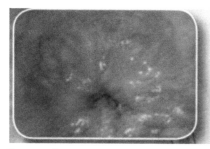 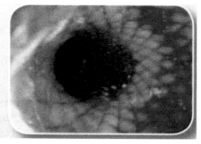

Fig. 1. Endoscopic result demonstrating dilation and placement of a covered stent allowing the passage of liquids and potentially some soft food. (Image courtesy Boston Scientific Endoscopy.)

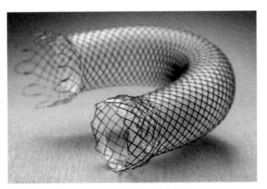

Fig. 2. Example of a self-expanding metal stent, with silicone coating. This product is available both as a fully- and partially covered prosthesis. (Image courtesy Boston Scientific Endoscopy.)

repositioning of the stent. Repositioning of the stent is less likely to be successful after the initial deployment, and if the stent has migrated too far, it will often need to be fully removed and a new stent deployed. The stents can be grasped with forceps through a flexible gastroscope and pulled out, by clamping onto the proximal string of the stent or the metal component of the stent itself. There is enough flexibility in the stent to allow this maneuver with a reasonable safety profile.

Most stents placed for obstruction will have a diameter of 18 mm. Larger stents of 23 mm are more useful in patients with tracheoesophageal fistula (TEF) or esophageal anastomotic leak. In those patients, a more occlusive stent is desirable.

Esophageal dilation and stenting can be performed under Monitored Anesthesia Care or General Anesthesia. In our experience, stenting is best accomplished with the patients intubated and under general anesthesia due to their aspiration morbidity associated with the obstructed patient. In addition, patients with upper-third or middle-third lesions will often need a bronchoscopy to assess the integrity of the airway as it pertains to tumor involvement, especially if CRT is to be considered as part of the palliative treatment plan.

SEMS can be deployed with fluoroscopic assist (**Fig. 3**) or by direct visualization, with the scope being positioned along the side of the stent, which has been advanced over a guidewire. The newest versions of through-the-scope "stents" are now being released, with a maximal diameter of 18 mm.

The deployment of the stent does not mean a resumption of a normal diet. Liquids, thick and thin, can be swallowed and so do most soft/moist or pureed foods. Counseling the patient on these limitations is very important, as it is not uncommon for a patient to return with a stent fully affected. Following stent placement these patients need a responsible provider who can answer questions and solve problems. Patients should be instructed what symptoms may occur with migration and who they should call if issues arrive. In an ideal situation when someone palliated with a stent develops acute recurrent dysphagia or nausea the response should not be "go to the local emergency room" but rather "let's get you into the office with a chest radiograph and see if the stent has migrated and remedy the situation."

Complications related to pain, obstruction, bleeding, migration, reflux, and erosion are well documented. If a patient is to proceed with palliative CRT, we recommend removal of the stents if the patient has achieved a documented clinical or radiographic response. Removal is usually achieved within 1 to 2 months of initiation of treatment. Rarely does the stent need to be replaced in the short term. Removal can prevent

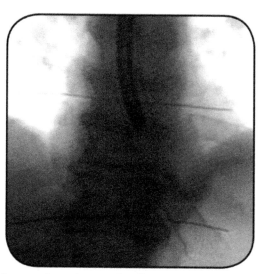

Fig. 3. Placement of an esophageal stent using fluoroscopy assistance. The stent is deployed under fluoroscopy with external radiopaque markers and final position verified by endoscopy. (Image courtesy Boston Scientific Endoscopy.)

some of the inherent complications of an indwelling stent, particularly migration and perforation.

Feeding tubes (gastric or jejunal) in conjunction with repetitive dilatation and CRT or endoluminal stenting may address the many early needs of a cachectic obstructed patient. With these forms of palliation in place, some patients have gone on to address their personal issues as it pertains to end of life planning and in many cases allow the patient to consider palliative CRT with subsequent response and survival measured in months or even years.

Doosti-Irani and colleagues[9] conducted an extensive review of published data and advanced statistical mapping to understand treatment-related complications from endoscopic stent placement. After an initial query of public literature of 17,855 references, 2017 were selected for review and 24 randomized controlled trials were retained for network analysis. Treatment-related complications included bleeding, stent migration, aspiration, pain, and fistula. Of the compared endoscopic therapies, thermal ablative therapy was associated with the least incidences of treatment-related complications, which was followed by covered stents and brachytherapy.

Kakuta and colleagues[5] published a retrospective review of 131 consecutive patients who underwent palliative intervention. Three groups were defined: endoscopic stenting, tube enterostomy for nutrition, and palliative esophagectomy. Key findings from this analysis include confirmation of the expectation that stenting would improve symptoms with no survival advantage. Interestingly, the complication rate of tube placement was very low but associated with a potential to improve survival due to the ability to improve nutrition and allow for additional treatments.

There are limited data comparing the efficacy and complications of palliative external beam radiation with esophageal stent placement. Martin and colleagues[10] aim to evaluate this question using a large database from the Veterans' Affairs. One thousand nine hundred fifty-seven (1957) veterans with metastatic esophageal cancer who received either palliative radiation or esophageal stenting were included. Of these 1593 underwent radiation and 364 underwent stenting. The cumulative incidence of any severe adverse effect at 6 months was higher among those who received stents compared with those who received radiation (21.7% vs 12.4%), with the most significant complications including fistula, perforation, and hemorrhage. Over time, it was believed that irradiation may have an advantage with similar long-term alleviation of dysphagia scores, although the immediate benefit to stenting in the short term must be considered. In a separate meta-analysis, it was established that stenting does not have to be isolated therapy, as the use of additional therapies in conjunction with stenting did not see an increase in complications.[11]

Brachytherapy may provide sustained relief; however, access to and availability of this technology is limited.[8] External beam radiation is more widely accessible, and stenting now has a track record of availability, immediate improvement of symptoms, and when provided as part of a multidisciplinary team is safe and effective.

Enteral Feeding Tubes

Nutrition and good hydration are an integral part of maintain health and well-being. In patients with locally advance esophageal cancer this is critical. Even in those patients who are successfully stented some patient may still need support via feeding tube. Tubes can be placed either in the stomach or in the small intestine. Both can be performed percutaneously or surgically. Feeding gastrostomy tubes have the advantage of bolus feeds, which can afford the patient avoidance of continuous or frequent feeding and pumps associated with jejunostomy. Also, they tend to be of larger caliber than jejunostomy tubes, and this results in less common occlusion. Gastrostomy tubes have disadvantages as well. For patients with stenting gastrostomy tubes may cause reflux, for patient with TEF reflux may result in aspiration into the airway. Gastrostomy tubes may also interfere with the creation of gastric conduit if the patient eventually comes to surgery. In the case of percutaneous gastrostomy tubes it may even damage the gastroepiploic artery precluding the use of the stomach for reconstruction.

Either gastrostomy or jejunostomy tubes can be successfully used in these patients. We frequently take advantage when a feeding tube is being placed to perform a staging laparoscopy simultaneously, and this can be very helpful in patients with locally advanced stage tumors.

Role of Surgery for Palliation

Before the era of effective endoscopic therapies, surgical resection was primarily offered for relief of the obstructive symptoms of esophageal cancer and to address the patient's nutritional needs. Ronald Belsey was fond of saying "resection and reconstruction for cancer of the esophagus is palliative, with an occasional cure." Although much has changed since that statement was made, as evident by the earlier articles in this book, for at least half of all patients diagnosed with esophageal cancer, much has not.

In the view of these investigators, palliative surgical resection is still an option in selective patients. In the absence of widely metastatic disease (ascites, carcinomatosis, etc.), resection can be performed for reasons of complete obstruction refractory to stenting, for esophageal perforation in the setting of stent placement gone awry, esophageal bleeding requiring multiple transfusions, or TEF.

In a patient presenting with TEF with a midesophageal squamous cell cancer, an esophageal isolation procedure is an option, with a pathologic segment of esophagus left in situ and the stomach pulled through a substernal space with a left neck anastomosis or in rare case going straight to spit fistula without reconstruction. Once recovered from surgery, the patient may then go on to CRT for treatment of the primary site of disease. Patient survival at times can be significantly prolonged with these interventions. When fistulas are left intact any treatment can make the fistula larger and speed up the patient's inevitable demise. Stenting is appealing but rarely fully occlusive and often requires double barrel technique (esophageal and tracheal stents placed simultaneously). Often the stent either fails to alleviate the symptoms of migration of enteral secretions into the airway or if successful it is short lived. On occasion the stent may actually exacerbate the issue by necrosing tumor. In some case an airway stent place for a fistula is retrieved a week later from the stomach. The ideal candidate for esophageal exclusion has a TEF without metastatic disease and without malnutrition. In our practice we meet many patients with TEF whom you prepare for the procedure only to find diffuse metastatic disease making any intervention useless. Operation for esophageal exclusion of TEF would only be recommended for locally advanced disease, without metastatic disease, and with expectation of survival beyond 3 or 4 months.

For complete obstruction or bleeding, a standard resection via abdominal only, abdomen/right chest approach (Ivor Lewis), or three-field approach (McKeown) would be the operations of choice and would include a feeding jejunostomy to enhance postoperative recovery. Other bypass techniques, in the absence of fistula, have also been described.[12]

Consensus Recommendations

In the 2020 European Journal of Cancer, a position statement was published[13] regarding the palliation of dysphagia in metastatic esophageal cancers. Key recommendations include multidisciplinary management with focus on nutritional support and quality-of-life measures. Endoscopic stenting should be considered in all patients with complete dysphagia, pending the implantation of other treatment or after failure, for infiltrating tumors less than 12 cm in length and at least 3 cm below the upper esophageal sphincter. In addition, front-line chemotherapy should be considered as directed by performance status, and radiation should be considered for patients who may have a life expectancy of longer than 3 months.

Future Directions

Advances in detection, diagnosis, staging, and therapeutics of esophageal cancer will fundamentally decrease the need for palliation. However, additional tools to assist in the care of a dying patient are under evaluation.

Yunqing Kang published a review article[14] that includes suggestion of intriguing future options that may be available to patients. All of these new technologies show promise but are not yet widely available and further studies will be required.

- Three-dimensional printed stents: additive manufacturing technologies may be used in conjunction with advanced imaging to provide customized prosthesis. This may offer a role in the future for personalized stents to optimize the patient's anatomy, while minimizing risk to surrounding structures including perforation and migration.
- Drug-eluting stents: self-expanding stents with a polymer membrane may allow for local delivery of cytotoxic agents, which may help with local tumor control, and minimize tumor growth.
- Biodegradable stents: the development of biodegradable polymer stents may help solve issues with tumor ingrowth, stent migration, and local erosion and fistula formation. The opportunity for local persistent dilatation and subsequent absorption of the stent material also obviates subsequent procedures for stent removal.

- Through-the-scope stents are increasingly available; however, their benefits over conventional stenting, which requires fluoroscopy, have yet to be realized.[15]

SUMMARY

- Esophageal cancer commonly presents in advanced stage, and many patients will require palliative intervention.
- Endoscopic stenting remains an excellent first-line therapy; however, this should be discussed in a multidisciplinary setting, taking in to account expectations for long-term survival and the risk of complications, which are time dependent, as a stent remains in place for longer periods.
- Provision of adequate nutrition is important and in patients with expectation for longer survival, tube enterostomy should be considered.
- Several investigational therapies show promise, most notably drug-eluting stent and biodegradable stents.

DISCLOSURE

The authors have nothing to disclose.

REFERENCES

1. Ferlay J, Shin HR, Bray F, et al. Estimates of worldwide burden of cancer in 2008: GLOBOCAN 2008. Int J Cancer 2010;127(12):2893–917.
2. Njei B, McCarty TR, Birk JW. Trends in esophageal cancer survival in United States adults from 1973 to 2009: a SEER database analysis. J Gastroenterol Hepatol 2016;31(6):1141–6.
3. Dunn GP. Surgical palliative care: recent trends and developments. Anesthesiol Clin 2012;30(1):13–28.
4. Halpern AL, McCarter MD. Palliative management of gastric and esophageal cancer. Surg Clin North Am 2019;99(3):555–69.
5. Kakuta T, Kosugi S-I, Ichikawa H, et al. Palliative interventions for patients with incurable locally advanced or metastatic thoracic esophageal carcinoma. Esophagus 2019;16(3):278–84.
6. van Rossum PSN, Mohammad NH, Vleggaar FP, et al. Treatment for unresectable or metastatic oesophageal cancer: current evidence and trends. Nat Rev Gastroenterol Hepatol 2018;15(4):235–49.
7. Lai A, Lipka S, Kumar A, et al. Role of esophageal metal stents placement and combination therapy in inoperable esophageal carcinoma: a systematic review and meta-analysis. Dig Dis Sci 2018;63(4):1025–34.
8. van der Bogt RD, Vermeulen BD, Reijm AN, et al. Palliation of dysphagia. Best Pract Res Clin Gastroenterol 2018;36-37:97–103.
9. Doosti-Irani A, Mansournia MA, Rahimi-Foroushani A, et al. Complications of stent placement in patients with esophageal cancer: a systematic review and network meta-analysis. PLoS One 2017;12(10):e0184784.
10. Martin EJ, Bruggeman AR, Nalawade VV, et al. Palliative radiotherapy versus esophageal stent placement in the management of patients with metastatic esophageal cancer. J Natl Compr Canc Netw 2020;18(5):569–74.
11. Tinusz B, Soós A, Hegyi P, et al. Efficacy and safety of stenting and additional oncological treatment versus stenting alone in unresectable esophageal cancer: a meta-analysis and systematic review. Radiother Oncol 2020;147:169–77.

12. Korst R. Surgical palliation of inoperable carcinoma of the esophagus. In: Shields TW, editor. General thoracic surgery. Lippincott Williams & Wilkins; 2005. Chapter 152 - Surgical Palliation of Inoperable Carcinoma of the Esophagus.

13. Levy A, Wagner AD, Chargari C, et al. Palliation of dysphagia in metastatic oesogastric cancers: an international multidisciplinary position. Eur J Cancer 2020; 135:103–12.

14. Kang Y. A review of self-expanding esophageal stents for the palliation therapy of inoperable esophageal malignancies. Biomed Res Int 2019;2019:9265017.

15. Vermeulen BD, Reijm AN, van der Bogt RD, et al. Through-the-scope placement of a fully covered metal stent for palliation of malignant dysphagia: a prospective cohort study (with video). Gastrointest Endosc 2019;90(6):972–9.

Surveillance Following Treatment of Esophageal Cancer

Charles T. Bakhos, MD, MS[a],*, Edwin Acevedo Jr, MD, MHA[b],
Roman V. Petrov, MD, PhD[a], Abbas E. Abbas, MD, MS[c]

KEYWORDS

- Neoadjuvant • Chemoradiation • Endoscopic resection • Salvage esophagectomy
- Outcomes

KEY POINTS

- Active surveillance of patients with esophageal cancer after chemoradiation can potentially allow organ preservation and reserve surgical resection to those with persistent disease or locoregional recurrence.
- Active surveillance also can be applied after local endoscopic therapy for early-stage esophageal cancer, with the goal of detecting early recurrence and allowing salvage treatment.
- There is currently no single imaging or invasive modality that can reliably detect persistent disease or locoregional recurrence after chemoradiation for esophageal cancer.
- Clinical Response Evaluation protocols incorporating a combination of different modalities can be implemented to optimize the accuracy of detecting esophageal cancer recurrence or persistent disease.
- Randomized clinical studies and more advanced imaging and/or invasive modalities are still necessary to justify the active surveillance of esophageal cancer that aim to defer surgical resection after chemoradiation.

INTRODUCTION

Esophageal cancer is currently the seventh leading cause of cancer-related mortality for men in the United States with a death rate of 3.9 per 100,000 men and women, claiming in total more than 18,000 lives.[1] Because of the lack of routine screening

[a] Department of Thoracic Medicine and Surgery, Lewis Katz School of Medicine, Temple University Hospital, 3401 North Broad Street C-501, Philadelphia, PA 19140, USA; [b] Department of Surgery, Temple University Hospital, 3401 North Broad Street C-501, Philadelphia, PA 19140, USA; [c] Department of Thoracic Medicine and Surgery, Lewis Katz School of Medicine, Temple University Hospital, Temple University Health System, 3401 North Broad Street C-501, Philadelphia, PA 19140, USA
* Corresponding author.
E-mail address: Charles.Bakhos@tuhs.temple.edu

Surg Clin N Am 101 (2021) 499–509
https://doi.org/10.1016/j.suc.2021.03.011
0039-6109/21/© 2021 Elsevier Inc. All rights reserved.

programs and frequently advanced stage at presentation, esophageal cancer is one of the most fatal malignancies with an overall 5-year survival rate of only 19.9%.[1] There are 2 main types of primary esophageal malignancies: squamous cell carcinoma (ESCC) and adenocarcinoma (EAC). These tumors differ in their risk factors, pathologic features, primary location, metastatic potential, and prognosis.[2] Treatment for esophageal cancer also differs based on histologic type and the degree of differentiation, as well as the clinical stage, genetic profile, and individual patient characteristics. Multidisciplinary evaluation is usually required to ensure the optimal treatment plan for each patient. Recent studies have demonstrated the survival benefit of the multimodality approach, establishing induction chemo or chemoradiation therapy (CRT) followed by surgical resection as a current standard of care for locoregional disease.[3–6] Despite these advancements, esophageal cancer frequently recurs with locoregional or distant disease, highlighting the importance of long-term surveillance.[3,7,8] Furthermore, up to 50% of patients with ESCC and 25% with EAC exhibit full pathologic response after CRT, prompting to question the value of added surgery with its associated morbidity and mortality.[3,5,9,10] This led to the concept of organ-preserving treatment, where surgery is offered after induction CRT only to patients with persistent disease or locoregional recurrence.[11,12] In fact, there is currently a phase III randomized Dutch trial (SANO: Surgery As Needed for Esophageal Cancer), aiming to compare the oncologic outcomes of neoadjuvant therapy with surgery as needed/active surveillance versus neoadjuvant therapy plus standard esophagectomy in patients with resectable EAC or ESCC.[13]

This paradigm shift is placing more emphasis on the surveillance strategy after esophageal cancer treatment, reserving surgery to a more select group of patients. In addition, advances in endoscopic treatment, such as endoscopic resection and even ablative techniques, have enabled esophageal sparing in very early stages of the disease.[14–17] In this context, surveillance to detect locoregional failure after organ-sparring esophageal cancer therapy is paramount to ensure oncologic outcomes that are comparable to traditional radical resection.

SURVEILLANCE AFTER NEOADJUVANT CHEMORADIOTHERAPY

In the early 1990s, the introduction of neoadjuvant chemoradiotherapy (nCRT) before surgery led to significant improvements in the rates of complete (R0) resection and in overall survival. This, however, was confounded by a trend toward increased early mortality in patients undergoing surgical resection.[18] Subsequent randomized controlled trials demonstrated that induction chemoradiation achieved pathologic complete response (pCR) in up to 50% of patients with squamous cell carcinoma, and in approximately 25% of those with adenocarcinoma of the esophagus.[5,19,20] In this setting, there is suggestion that patients could undergo active surveillance to detect locoregional recurrence with similar overall survival when compared with planned esophagectomy. For instance, a retrospective review of 77 patients with ESCC who underwent nCRT compared the outcomes of those who proceeded with esophagectomy (n = 39) with those who either refused surgery or were thought to be unfit for it (n = 38). The 5-year overall survival and 5-year disease-free survival were comparable between the trimodality group and nCRT group (50% vs 57%, 55.5% vs 34.6%, respectively). Even after adjusting for propensity score, age, American Society of Anesthesiologists class and clinical stage, there was no significant difference in these 2 outcome measures.[21] Another large retrospective series of patients with esophagogastric cancer from MD Anderson Cancer Center showed comparable findings. In a cohort of 623 patients, 244 patients underwent trimodality therapy (TMT) and 61 patients who were eligible for surgery after nCRT did decline it. Using the propensity score method, the investigators matched 16 covariates between 36 patients who underwent TMT and 36 patients who declined surgery. The median overall survival times was 50.8 months for the TMT group and 57.9 months for the patients who just underwent nCRT ($P = .28$). The median relapse-free survival was 26.5 months and 18.5 months ($P = .45$), respectively. Of note though is that 11 (31%) of the 36 patients who had declined surgery later underwent salvage resection.[22] These 2 studies are retrospective in nature and have many limitations, including a relatively small number of patients and an inherent selection bias despite the propensity score analysis. Although no firm conclusions can be drawn from them, they do suggest that an active surveillance strategy after nCRT could capture locoregional recurrences and prompt surgical resection without a significant impact on overall survival.

In that context, it is crucial to identify a pathologic complete response (pCR) and define the active surveillance strategy. A pathologic complete response is classically depicted on the post-resection surgical specimen; in the clinical context that does not include surgery, pCR constitutes no tumor detection on clinical response evaluations (CREs). The latter has been proposed in the Netherlands to distinguish complete clinical response (cCR) to nCRT from those with residual disease while it is still resectable, in patients with esophageal cancer undergoing the Cincinnati Research in Outcomes and Safety in Surgery (CROSS) regimen.[12] CREs should precede active surveillance, and typically involve a combination of diagnostic modalities to increase the accuracy, sensitivity, and specificity of detection.[20] Active surveillance is initiated after confirmation of cCR to nCRT and should be regularly performed at specific time intervals to capture locoregional or distant recurrence, so salvage resection or additional chemoradiotherapy can be offered in a timely fashion.

Current active surveillance modalities include various imaging techniques and invasive procedures, such as computed tomography (CT), PET-CT, MRI, endoscopy, and endoscopic ultrasound (EUS). The value and accuracy of these modalities vary, and care must be taken to select the most appropriate study for the diagnostic purpose. As we discuss in the following, a combination of these modalities is often required to increase the diagnostic yield.

Residual or Recurrent Locoregional Disease after Neoadjuvant Chemoradiotherapy

Esophagogastroduodenoscopy (EGD) is an essential component of the initial evaluation of patients with suspected esophageal cancer, allowing tissue sampling via mucosal biopsies. Its role in surveillance after nCRT is, however, more questionable, mostly due to the resulting mucosal inflammation. A recent meta-analysis of 12 studies comprising a total of 1328 patients evaluated endoscopic biopsies for detecting any residual disease at the primary tumor site.[23] Sensitivity and specificity of positive versus negative biopsies ranged from 0.11 to 0.59 and from 0.77 to 1.00, respectively, reflecting significant heterogeneity among these studies. The pooled sensitivity was 0.33 and pooled specificity 0.95. Of note that 3 studies were prospective, and only 2 reported the number of biopsies (median of 4). It is also important to mention 2 issues when discussing the role of EGD with biopsy in the post-neoadjuvant setting. The first is the type of biopsy that is being performed. A pre-SANO trial demonstrated that bite-on-bite biopsies increased the chance of detecting residual cancer cells in deeper layers of the esophagus, such as the submucosa, compared with regular biopsies.[24] The second is the interpretation of pathologic data. In the same study, at least 2 independent expert pathologists reviewed each endoscopic and surgical specimen, and their learning curve seemed to improve over time based on strict protocols. This being said, EGD with biopsy still exhibits a substantially high false negative rate, and therefore is not considered a reliable single modality to evaluate clinical response and detect residual esophageal wall cancer after nCRT.

EUS plays a significant role in the initial staging of esophageal cancer, and in general is considered to be superior to CT scan in evaluating the depth of tumor invasion (accuracy of 76%–89% vs 49%–59%, respectively).[25] In the post-neoadjuvant setting, EUS can be used to detect residual esophageal wall disease, and to assess for persistent lymph node (LN) metastasis though fine needle aspiration (FNA). The sensitivity and specificity of this modality are obscured by the usual inflammatory changes that are observed after chemoradiation, however. The timing of EUS and other surveillance modality is important in this context, as the inflammation tends to subside after 12 weeks from the end of CRT. In clinical practice though, it recommended that surgery is performed within 6 to 8 weeks of the end of CRT to optimize the outcomes, although this concept is being challenged.[26] Regarding the accuracy of posttreatment EUS, a recent meta-analysis by Eyck and colleagues[23] found a pooled sensitivity and specificity for the detection of residual cancer at the primary tumor site of 96% and 8%, respectively. Among the included studies (n = 11), 42.8% of patients had ESCC, and the intervals between the end of nCRT and EUS ranged from less than 14 days to 42 days. There was also significant heterogeneity among the studies, reflecting the operator dependency in endosonographic techniques. The overall positive predictive value (PPV) was 0.67 and negative predictive value (NPV) was 0.51, reflecting the challenge of using EUS solely to detect residual cancer on a case-by-case basis. The pooled sensitivity of qualitative EUS to detect residual nodal disease was 0.68 (range 0.26–0.94) and the pooled specificity 0.57 (range 0.23–1.00). Of note was that only one study reported using FNA to sample the LNs. More clinically relevant though, the underlying histology seems to influence the accuracy of EUS in detecting residual LN metastasis. The sensitivity of EUS in studies that had more than 80% squamous cell carcinomas was better (0.81) compared with the studies that had more than 80% adenocarcinomas (0.52), whereas the specificity was worse (0.52 vs 0.68, respectively).

CT is usually helpful in the initial staging of esophageal cancer, mainly through the detection of regional LNs and distant metastasis. Its role in assessing the initial T stage is quite limited to begin with, as the abnormal esophageal wall thickness >5 mm is nonspecific.[27] Even the obliteration of fat planes between the esophagus and adjacent structures, a characteristic CT finding of a T4 tumor, is nonspecific and can occur in patients with prior radiation.[25] CT is more accurate in demonstrating enlarged regional lymph nodes, but the specificity for metastases is suboptimal. In a meta-analysis of 17 studies, the pooled sensitivity and specificity in detecting regional lymph node metastasis in the initial staging was 50% and 83%, respectively.[28] There are currently very limited data on the usefulness of CT scan following neoadjuvant treatment, and physicians rely more on combined CT-PET modality in the clinical response evaluation.

PET-CT is a very valuable tool in the initial staging of esophageal cancer, particularly for the evaluation of regional and distant disease. Following neoadjuvant treatment, the PET scan information can be interpreted from a qualitative perspective in terms of metabolic response, and a quantitative perspective in terms of percentage change in the Standard Uptake Value (%ΔSUVmax). Unfortunately, a confounding factor that affects the degree of uptake is the inflammation due to radiation, esophagitis, worsening reflux, or combination of these. Comparable to EGD and EUS-FNA data, analyzing the PET-CT literature in the post-neoadjuvant setting should be done carefully, as most studies are retrospective, often lack statistical power, and more importantly are not necessarily designed to detect residual disease and distinguish who would benefit from surveillance versus surgical resection. A recent meta-analysis of

14 studies reported qualitative PET results as complete metabolic response or non-complete metabolic response at the primary tumor site.[23] The pooled sensitivity was 0.74 (95% confidence interval [CI] 0.68–0.79) and the pooled specificity 0.52 (95% CI 0.44–0.60). The same meta-analysis included 7 studies (n = 511 patients) that reported quantitative percentage reduction in SUVmax, with a median cutoff of 72.3% (range 52%–79.3%). The pooled sensitivity was comparable at 0.73, but the pooled specificity improved at 0.63. More importantly and from a clinically relevant perspective, the sensitivity was significantly higher in studies that included more than 80% squamous cell carcinomas versus more than 80% adenocarcinomas (0.8 vs 0.43). Other limitations of PET-CT that have been highlighted in another preSANO side study is the lack of accuracy in detecting tumor regression grade, and the inability to distinguish relapse from inflammation up to 12 weeks after nCRT.[29] This being said, PET-CT should not be overlooked after nCRT, as it can help detect distant disease, as we discuss next.

Distant Metastasis after Neoadjuvant Chemoradiotherapy

Accurate detection of disease progression and distant metastasis in esophageal cancer after nCRT cannot be overemphasized for avoidance of the futile noncurative surgical resection. In fact, up to 5% to 10% of patients will develop distant metastases after induction therapy.[5,30] In a large case-series of 783 patients, 65 (8.3%) were found to have interval metastasis on PET-CT, and 44 (5.6%) were deemed to have false positive lesions. The overall sensitivity and specificity of PET-CT were 74.7% and 93.7%, respectively.[31] Multivariate analysis revealed that tumor length, clinical nodal status, squamous cell tumor histology, and baseline SUVmax were associated with a higher risk of interval metastasis. The issue of false positives in this setting was also demonstrated in another retrospective study of 205 patients, which reported 6 cases (3%) of radiation-induced metabolically active liver lesions mimicking metastases.[32] A recent meta-analysis of 14 studies comprising a total of 1110 patients showed similar findings, with an 8% rate of interval metastases and 5% incidence of false positive.[30] These studies highlight the importance of PET-CT after nCRT in avoiding unnecessary and noncurative surgery, but also the need for tissue confirmation of suspected metastatic lesions.

In summary, the clinical response evaluation and active surveillance of resectable esophageal cancer after nCRT is important to determine the need for surgical resection. Review of the literature shows that EGD with biopsy, EUS (with FNA), CT scan, and PET-CT are insufficiently accurate in isolation to detect residual disease and locoregional recurrence. PET-CT can be very valuable to detect interval metastasis, but necessitates tissue confirmation due to a non-negligible incidence of false positives. The evaluation for relapse or disease progression should therefore involve a multimodal approach that is adapted to each clinical scenario.

SURVEILLANCE AFTER DEFINITIVE CHEMORADIOTHERAPY

The concept of definitive chemoradiotherapy (dCRT), or chemoradiotherapy without surgery for esophageal cancer is not new, and has been successfully applied to other malignancies.[33,34] In patients with esophageal cancer, definitive chemoradiotherapy has been typically reserved for patients with unresectable, locally advanced disease (ie, stage T4b), or patients with poor physical reserve that precludes surgical resection. Timing and imaging modality for surveillance in patients with locally aggressive disease that undergo dCRT remains under investigation, but surveillance is required to ensure good response to therapy and to detect residual or recurrent disease that would enable the implementation of salvage therapies, such as additional chemotherapy and/or radiation therapy, or even surgical resection. Salvage esophagectomy is discussed at greater length in another article in this issue.

Surveillance in this setting typically uses a combination of the modalities we discussed earlier, to detect recurrence or disease progression. At our institution, we perform an EGD every 4 months during the first year, then every 6 months thereafter. We also obtain a contrast CT scan of the chest, abdomen, and pelvis every 6 months for the first 3 years, and a PET scan at the end of the first year and then as needed. The surveillance modality naturally adapts to each patient's needs and postoperative imaging or endoscopic findings.

SURVEILLANCE AFTER ENDOSCOPIC TREATMENT OF EARLY-STAGE ESOPHAGEAL CANCER

Endoscopic management of esophageal cancer has gained in popularity in the past decade, as another organ-sparing modality in early-stage disease with low likelihood of LN spread, such as mucosal (T1a) esophageal adenocarcinoma. Endoscopic treatment even has been suggested as a reasonable alternative to esophagectomy for T1b submucosal EAC with certain favorable features and in patients who are suboptimal surgical candidates. These include tumors with less than 500-μm invasion in the submucosa [sm1], good to moderate differentiation, and no lymphatic invasion.[35] Of note is that the risk of LN metastasis seems to be higher in early-stage ESCC compared with EAC, as shown in a retrospective review of 7645 resected specimens.[35] Endoscopic techniques in this setting include a variety of resection and ablation modalities, such as endoscopic mucosal resection (EMR), endoscopic submucosal dissection (ESD), radiofrequency ablation, cryotherapy, and photodynamic therapy, to name a few. Naturally, the main concern in endoscopic management of early-stage esophageal cancer is local recurrence, justifying frequent endoscopic surveillance in most studies comparing local therapy with traditional esophagectomy. In an early report from the Mayo Clinic comparing EMR (n = 132) and surgery (n = 46) for stage T1a mucosal EAC, Prasad and colleagues[36] showed no significant difference in overall survival between the 2 groups, at a mean follow-up period of 64 months. Rigorous endoscopic surveillance after local endoscopic treatment was performed, detecting 16 (12%) recurrences at an average of 19 months after initial treatment. These recurrences were subsequently successfully treated with repeat EMR in all but 1 patient who opted for esophagectomy.[36] Another comparative study of 114 patients with mucosal adenocarcinoma showed no difference in survival between transthoracic esophageal resection with 2 field lymphadenectomy (n = 38) and endoscopic resection (n = 76). The latter included endoscopic resection followed by argon plasma coagulation of the remaining nondysplastic Barrett esophagus.[14] The surveillance regimen in this study was quite rigorous, and included endoscopic examination at 1, 2, 3, 6, 9, and 12 months after treatment and then at 6-month intervals up to the end of a 5-year period after treatment. The check-ups included endoscopy with high-resolution endoscopes and biopsies of any suspicious lesions, as well as 4-quadrant biopsies and/or chromoendoscopy of residual Barrett mucosa. At a median follow-up of 4.1 years in the endoscopic resection group, 1 patient had a local recurrence and 4 had metachronous tumors (overall recurrence rate 6.6%), all of whom underwent repeat endoscopic treatment.

These studies highlight the value of endoscopic surveillance in detecting recurrences after the local treatment of early-stage esophageal cancer. Current recommendations are to proceed with EGD and biopsies after endoscopic therapy of early-stage EAC at 3, 6, and 12 months and annual intervals, with emphasis on using high-definition white-light endoscopy, careful inspection of the neosquamous mucosa, and performance of retroflexion inspection of the gastric cardia.[37] This regimen should be altered according to patients' characteristics, tumor features, and resection/ablation technical factors. In that regard, a systematic review of endoscopic resection of early-stage esophageal carcinoma, local tumor recurrence was best predicted by grade 3 differentiation, piecemeal resection, metachronous cancer development in the carcinoma in situ component, and lymphovascular invasion. Piecemeal resection, a proxy for positive margin, was more common in EMR as opposed to the ESD technique.[38]

FUTURE DIRECTIONS

Despite significant progress in the diagnosis and staging of esophageal cancer, there is no single modality that can reliably detect local recurrence or residual disease with a clinically acceptable degree of accuracy. As discussed earlier, surveillance after esophageal cancer treatment does in practice require diagnostic vigilance through a combination of the available modalities to address individual clinical scenarios. There are new technologies on the horizon, however, that can potentially address the need for more accurate diagnosis of locoregional and distant recurrences during the active surveillance of esophageal cancer.

Magnetic Resonance Imaging

MRI has the advantage of avoiding ionizing radiation and has significantly better spatial resolution than PET-CT and CT. Whole-body MRI has been compared with PET-CT in the initial staging of esophageal cancer in a prospective study of 49 patients, and showed similar accuracy in detecting nodal deposits and metastatic disease.[39] High-resolution (HR) MRI was also found to be superior to conventional MRI in the initial staging of 118 patients with pathologically confirmed gastroesophageal junction malignancies.[40] Specifically, there was better agreement in the T1 stage between the pathologic specimen and HR-MRI. However, both imaging techniques were comparable in differentiating the T stages of $\leq$ T1 from $\geq$ T2 and the T stages of $\leq$ T3 from $\geq$ T4. There is a relative paucity of data regarding the value of MRI in the neoadjuvant setting. A report by Heethuis and colleagues[41] showed promising results of dynamic contrast-enhanced (DCE) MRI in predicting histopathological response, in a series of 26 patients who underwent the study before, during (week 2–3), and after nCRT but before surgery. Comparison of tumor area under the concentration time curve before and after treatment was most predictive for complete pathologic response, with a sensitivity of 83%, specificity of 88%, PPV of 71%, and an NPV of 93%. The MRI findings were compared with the resected surgical specimens in this study. Another recent study by Vollenbrock and colleagues[42] investigated the diagnostic performance of visual response assessment of the primary tumor after nCRT on T2-weighted (T2W) and diffusion-weighted (DW) MRI. In a series of 51 patients, 3 radiologists independently and blindly evaluated T2W images using a 5-point score for the assessment of residual tumor and immediately rescored after adding DW-MRI. Histopathology of the resection specimen was used as the reference standard in this retrospective study, with 12 patients showing a complete pathologic response. The sensitivity of T2W + DW-MRI for detecting residual tumor was 90% to 97%, but the specificity was 42% to 50% only, potentially overstaging complete responder as having residual disease. In addition, the interrater reliability (κ value) was rather weak to moderate, and ranged from 0.24 to 0.55 on T2W-MRI to 0.55 to 0.71 with DW-MRI.[42] A subsequent study of 33 patients by the same group compared DW-MRI with PET-CT in assessing the clinical response after nCRT, and demonstrated a higher diagnostic accuracy for the detection of residual tumor (71% vs 54%) and nodal disease (89% vs 75%).[43] The specificity for the 2 individual readers to detect local disease on DW-MRI was still relatively low, and ranged from 43% to 57%.

In practice, the application of MRI technology after neoadjuvant treatment for esophageal cancer remains limited to a few quaternary centers and/or clinical trial protocols. Slower image acquisition in comparison with CT and PET-CT, interobserver disagreement, and readers' learning curve remain obstacles against the widespread adoption of this imaging technology.

Circulating Tumor DNA in Plasma

Many of the surveillance strategies involve imaging or invasive procedures, each with their respective risks and benefits. These disadvantages have created a clinical need for biomarkers that can be obtained with minimal risk to the patient. Circulating tumor DNA (ctDNA) is a promising new biomarker that is currently under investigation. The presence of ctDNA in the plasma of patients with cancer is well-established.[44–46] Studies have attempted to detect and quantify stage-specific differences in ctDNA in esophageal adenocarcinoma, and the results are promising. In the evaluation of 38 patients with esophageal adenocarcinoma, 18 (47%) patients demonstrated positive ctDNA. More importantly, the levels increased with the tumor burden and preceded recurrence.[47] Comparable results were found in another recent study of 45 patients who underwent deep sequencing analyses of plasma cell-free DNA before and after chemoradiotherapy for esophageal cancer. Detection of ctDNA after CRT was associated with tumor progression, formation of distant metastases, and shorter disease-specific survival times. Furthermore, a higher proportion of patients with tumor progression had new mutations detected in plasma samples collected after CRT than patients without progression.[48] The ability to detect ctDNA in all patients remains challenging, however, as they are usually found in minute quantities and require special handling and processing.[47,48] Ideally, ctDNA would be used to detect early cancer, assess treatment response, detect the presence of residual tumor, and identify treatment failure. Although this "liquid biopsy" is a promising new development that may eventually provide prognostic information in the management of esophageal cancer, further investigation is necessary to validate its clinical application.

SUMMARY

Much progress has been made in the treatment of esophageal cancer with the introduction of new chemoradiation regimens that have positively improved outcomes. Although CRT followed by surgery remains the standard of care for locoregional esophageal cancer and is the preferred management in our practice, current diagnostic modalities allow for earlier detection and more accurate staging of the disease. These advances have made organ preservation feasible via endoscopic resection techniques that do not necessarily jeopardize long-term survival. Even surgery-sparing protocols have been developed after nCRT, with the goal of avoiding the morbidity of esophagectomy. Active surveillance in these settings is paramount in the management of esophageal cancer, for the accurate detection of persistent disease or early recurrence, to allow salvage intervention. Currently, there is no single imaging or testing modality that can reliably detect persistent disease or locoregional recurrence. Rather, a combination of the imaging and invasive modalities is required for timely detection of treatment failures. New technologies, such as DCE-MRI and biomarker/DNA testing, are currently under investigation, and may be beneficial for the early detection of relapse after esophageal cancer treatment.

DISCLOSURE

The authors have no disclosures.

REFERENCES

1. National Cancer Institute. Cancer stat facts: esophageal cancer. SEER Cancer Statistics Review. 2019. 2019. Available at: https://seer.cancer.gov/statfacts/html/esoph.html. Accessed August 20, 2020.
2. Mariette C, Finzi L, Piessen G, et al. Esophageal carcinoma: prognostic differences between squamous cell carcinoma and adenocarcinoma. World J Surg 2005;29(1):39–45.
3. Shapiro J, van Lanschot J, Hulshof M, et al. Neoadjuvant chemoradiotherapy plus surgery versus surgery alone for oesophageal or junctional cancer (CROSS): long-term results of a randomised controlled trial. Lancet Oncol 2015;16(9): 1090–8.
4. Cunningham D, Allum W, Stenning S, et al. Perioperative chemotherapy versus surgery for resectable gastroesophageal cancer. N Engl J Med 2006;355(1): 11–20.
5. Van Hagen P, Hulshof MC, van Lanschot JJ, et al. Preoperative chemoradiotherapy for esophageal or junctional cancer. N Engl J Med 2012;366(22):2074–84.
6. Steffen T, Dietrich D, Schnider A, et al. Recurrence patterns and long-term results after induction chemotherapy, chemoradiotherapy, and curative surgery in patients with locally advanced esophageal cancer. Ann Surg 2019;269(1):83–7.
7. Barbetta A, Sihag S, Nobel T, et al. Patterns and risk of recurrence in patients with esophageal cancer with a pathologic complete response after chemoradiotherapy followed by surgery. J Thorac Cardiovasc Surg 2019;157(3):1249–59.e5.
8. Lou F, Sima CS, Adusumilli PS, et al. Esophageal cancer recurrence patterns and implications for surveillance. J Thorac Oncol 2013;8(12):1558–62.
9. Klevebro F, Alexandersson von Döbeln G, Wang N, et al. A randomized clinical trial of neoadjuvant chemotherapy versus neoadjuvant chemoradiotherapy for cancer of the oesophagus or gastro-oesophageal junction. Ann Oncol 2016; 27(4):660–7.
10. Yang H, Liu H, Chen Y, et al. Neoadjuvant Chemoradiotherapy Followed by Surgery versus Surgery Alone for Locally Advanced Squamous Cell Carcinoma of the Esophagus (NEOCRTEC5010): a Phase III multicenter, randomized, open-label clinical trial. J Clin Oncol 2018;36(27):2796–803.
11. Semenkovich TR, Meyers B. Surveillance versus esophagectomy in esophageal cancer patients with a clinical complete response after induction chemoradiation. Ann Transl Med 2018;6(4):81.
12. Van der Wilk BJ, Eyck BM, Spaander MCW, et al. Towards an organ-sparing approach for locally advanced esophageal cancer. Dig Surg 2019;36(6):462–9.
13. Noordman BJ, Wijnhoven BPL, Lagarde SM, et al. Neoadjuvant chemoradiotherapy plus surgery versus active surveillance for oesophageal cancer: a stepped-wedge cluster randomized trial. BMC Cancer 2018;18(1):142.
14. Pech O, Bollschweiler E, Manner H, et al. Comparison between endoscopic and surgical resection of mucosal esophageal adenocarcinoma in Barrett's esophagus at two high-volume centers. Ann Surg 2011;254(1):67–72.
15. Shaheen N, Sharma P, Overholt B, et al. Radiofrequency ablation in Barrett's esophagus with dysplasia. N Engl J Med 2009;360(22):2277–88.
16. Haidry RJ, Butt MA, Dunn JM, et al. Improvement over time in outcomes for patients undergoing endoscopic therapy for Barrett's oesophagus-related

neoplasia: 6-year experience from the first 500 patients treated in the UK patient registry. Gut 2015;64(8):1192–9.

17. Pech O, May A, Manner H, et al. Long-term efficacy and safety of endoscopic resection for patients with mucosal adenocarcinoma of the esophagus. Gastroenterology 2014;146(3):652–60.

18. Urschel J, Vasan H, Blewett C. A meta-analysis of randomized controlled trials that compared neoadjuvant chemotherapy and surgery to surgery alone for resectable esophageal cancer. Am J Surg 2002;183(3):274–9.

19. de Gouw DJJM, Klarenbeek BR, Driessen M, et al. Detecting pathological complete response in esophageal cancer after neoadjuvant therapy based on imaging techniques: a diagnostic systematic review and meta-analysis. J Thorac Oncol 2019;14(7):1156–71.

20. Noordman BJ, Spaander M, Valkema R, et al. Detection of residual disease after neoadjuvant chemoradiotherapy for oesophageal cancer (PreSANO): a prospective multicenter, diagnostic cohort study. Lancet Oncol 2018;19(7):965–74.

21. Castoro C, Scarpa M, Cagol M, et al. Complete clinical response after neoadjuvant chemoradiotherapy for squamous cell cancer of the thoracic oesophagus: is surgery always necessary? J Gastrointest Surg 2013;17:1375–81.

22. Taketa T, Xiao L, Sudo K. Propensity-based matching between esophagogastric cancer patients who had surgery and who declined surgery after preoperative chemoradiation. Oncology 2013;85(2):95–9.

23. Eyck BM, Onstenk BD, Noordman BJ, et al. Accuracy of detecting residual disease after neoadjuvant chemoradiotherapy for esophageal cancer a systematic review and meta-analysis. Ann Surg 2020;271(2):245–56.

24. Noordman BJ, Shapiro J, Spaander MC, et al. Accuracy of detecting residual disease after cross neoadjuvant chemoradiotherapy for esophageal cancer (PRESANO trial): rationale and protocol. JMIR Res Protoc 2015;4(2):e79.

25. Napier K. Esophageal cancer: a review of epidemiology, pathogenesis, staging workup and treatment modalities. World J Gastroint Oncol 2014;6(5):112.

26. Levinsky NC, Wima K, Morris MC, et al. Cincinnati Research in Outcomes and Safety in Surgery (CROSS) Group. Outcome of delayed versus timely esophagectomy after chemoradiation for esophageal adenocarcinoma. J Thorac Cardiovasc Surg 2020;159(6):2555–66.

27. Desai RK, Tagliabue JR, Wegryn S, et al. CT evaluation of wall thickening in the alimentary tract. Radiographics 1991;11(5):771–83 [discussion: 784].

28. Van Vliet EP, Van Heijenbrok-Kal MH, Hunink M, et al. Staging investigations for oesophageal cancer: a meta-analysis. Br J Cancer 2008;98(3):547–57.

29. Valkema MJ, Noordman BJ, Wijnhoven BPL, et al. Accuracy of 18F-FDG PET/CT in predicting residual disease after neoadjuvant chemoradiotherapy for esophageal cancer. J Nucl Med 2019;60(11):1553–9.

30. Kroese TE, Goense L, van Hillegersberg R, et al. Detection of distant interval metastases after neoadjuvant therapy for esophageal cancer with 18 F-FDG PET(/CT): a systematic review and meta-analysis. Dis Esophagus 2018;31(12):1–9.

31. Goense L, Ruurda JP, Carter BW, et al. Prediction and diagnosis of interval metastasis after neoadjuvant chemoradiotherapy for oesophageal cancer using 18 F-FDG PET/CT. Eur J Nucl Med Mol Imaging 2018;45:1742–51.

32. Voncken FEM, Aleman B, van Dieren J, et al. Radiation-induced liver injury mimicking liver metastases on FDG-PET-CT after chemoradiotherapy for esophageal cancer: a retrospective study and literature review. Strahlenther Onkol 2018; 194(2):156–63.

33. Zenda S, Kojima T, Kato K, et al. Multicenter phase 2 study of cisplatin and 5-fluorouracil with concurrent radiation therapy as an organ preservation approach in patients with squamous cell carcinoma of the cervical esophagus. Int J Radiat Oncol Biol Phys 2016;96(5):976–84.

34. De Felice F, Martinetti M, Orelli S, et al. Definitive chemoradiotherapy for anal carcinoma: long-term results based on consistent time-to-event endpoints. Oncology 2018;94(1):25–30.

35. Gockel I, Sgourakis G, Lyros O, et al. Risk of lymph node metastasis in submucosal esophageal cancer: a review of surgically resected patients. Rev Expert Rev Gastroenterol Hepatol 2011;5(3):371–84.

36. Prasad G, Wu T, Wigle D, et al. Endoscopic and surgical treatment of mucosal (T1a) esophageal adenocarcinoma in Barrett's esophagus. Gastroenterology 2009;137(3):815–23.

37. Sharma P, Shaheen N, Katzka D, et al. AGA clinical practice update on endoscopic treatment of barrett's esophagus with dysplasia and/or early cancer: expert review. Gastroenterology 2020;158(3):760–9.

38. Sgourakis G, Gockel I, Lang H. Endoscopic and surgical resection of T1a/T1b esophageal neoplasms: a systematic review. World J Gastroenterol 2013;19(9): 1424–37.

39. Malik V, Harmon M, Johnston C, et al. Whole body MRI in the staging of esophageal cancer - a prospective comparison with whole body 18F-FDG PET-CT. Dig Surg 2015;32:397–408.

40. Yuan Y, Chen L, Ren S, et al. Diagnostic performance in T staging for patients with esophagogastric junction cancer using high-resolution MRI: a comparison with conventional MRI at 3 Tesla. Cancer Imaging 2019;19(1):83.

41. Heethuis SE, van Rossum PS, Lips IM, et al. Dynamic contrast-enhanced MRI for treatment response assessment in patients with oesophageal cancer receiving neoadjuvant chemoradiotherapy. Radiother Oncol 2016;120(1):128–35.

42. Vollenbrock S, Voncken FEM, Van Dieren J, et al. Diagnostic performance of MRI for assessment of response to neoadjuvant chemoradiotherapy in oesophageal cancer. Br J Surg 2019;106(5):596–605.

43. Vollenbrock SE, Voncken FEM, Lambregts DMJ, et al. Clinical response assessment on DW-MRI compared with FDG-PET/CT after neoadjuvant chemoradiotherapy in patients with oesophageal cancer. Eur J Nucl Med Mol Imaging 2020. https://doi.org/10.1007/s00259-020-04917-5.

44. Bettegowda C, Sausen M, Leary R, et al. Detection of circulating tumor DNA in early- and late-stage human malignancies. Sci Transl Med 2014;6(224):224ra24.

45. Cohen J, Li L, Wang Y, et al. Detection and localization of surgically resectable cancers with a multi-analyte blood test. Cancer 2018;359:926–30.

46. Borggreve AS, Mook S, Verheij M, et al. Preoperative image-guided identification of response to neoadjuvant chemoradiotherapy in esophageal cancer (PRIDE): a multicenter observational study. BMC Cancer 2018;18(1):1006.

47. Egyud M, Tejani M, Pennathur A, et al. Detection of circulating tumor DNA in plasma: a potential biomarker for esophageal adenocarcinoma. Ann Thorac Surg 2019;108(2):343–9.

48. Azad TD, Chaudhuri AA, Fang P, et al. Circulating tumor DNA analysis for detection of minimal residual disease after chemoradiotherapy for localized esophageal cancer. Gastroenterology 2020;158(3):494–505.

Techniques of Esophageal Anastomoses for Esophagectomy

Robert Herron, DO, Ghulam Abbas, MD, MHCM*

KEYWORDS

- Esophagectomy • Esophagogastric anastomosis
- Techniques of esophageal anastomosis • Minimally invasive esophagectomy
- Robotic-assisted minimally invasive esophagectomy

KEY POINTS

- Various techniques in the creation of the esophagogastric anastomosis in esophagectomy are discussed.
- The performance of an anastomotic technique can be surgeon specific, although it is of great benefit for the esophageal surgeon to be facile and adept in multiple techniques as occasionally the clinical situation may be better suited for a particular technique.
- Regardless of the method of creating the esophagogastric anastomosis, the goal is to create a viable, tension-free and nonobstructive anastomosis with adequate margins.

INTRODUCTION

Esophageal cancer continues to be a highly fatal malignancy, preferentially affecting men, and ranks as the sixth most common cause of cancer-related mortality worldwide.[1]

The Western world, to include North America, Europe, and Australia, has seen a surge in esophageal adenocarcinoma due to lifestyle-associated risk factors such as gastroesophageal reflux disease, obesity, and Barrett esophagus. Esophagectomy for the treatment of esophageal cancer was described more than a century ago with historically poor survival. The operative approach for esophagectomy has revolutionized over the past 3 decades, first with the advent of minimally invasive surgery and recently with the introduction of robotic-assisted surgery. Similarly, the overall survival has significantly improved due to more accurate preoperative staging, better patient selection, introduction of neoadjuvant treatment, and improved postoperative care. More accurate preoperative staging is accomplished due to the easy availability of PET-computed tomography (CT), as well as endoscopic ultrasound. This aids in selecting patients

Division of Thoracic Surgery, Department of Thoracic and Cardiovascular Surgery, West Virginia University, WVU School of Medicine, 1 Medical Center Drive, Morgantown, WV 26506, USA
* Corresponding author.
E-mail address: ghulam.abbas@hsc.wvu.edu

Surg Clin N Am 101 (2021) 511–524
https://doi.org/10.1016/j.suc.2021.03.012
0039-6109/21/© 2021 Elsevier Inc. All rights reserved.
surgical.theclinics.com

who will benefit from induction treatment. The landmark MAGIC and FLOT trials showed that the utilization of neoadjuvant chemotherapy followed by esophagectomy led to a 5-year survival of 36% and 45% respectively.[2,3] Similarly, the CROSS trial has shown significant improvement in overall and disease-free survival with the addition of chemoradiation as neoadjuvant treatment.[4] Even a century after its description, esophagectomy is considered to be one of the most complex surgical interventions performed on the gastrointestinal tract and it continues to evolve and improve. There are various techniques for surgical resection of the esophagus. These techniques include traditional open approaches and minimally invasive approaches, including robotic-assisted techniques. Ultimately the procedure culminates in an anastomosis between the esophagus and the conduit in either the cervical or intrathoracic location. These variations address several factors that include the patient, location of the tumor, the size of tumor, tumor margins, and surgeon's preferences.

This article describes the various techniques of esophagectomy with an emphasis on the techniques of creating the esophagogastric anastomosis.

PRINCIPLES OF ESOPHAGECTOMY

The anatomy of the esophagus is complex in that it is in close proximity to many vital structures within the chest: the trachea, right and left mainstem bronchi, the pericardium, azygous vein, the aorta, and the diaphragm. Should an esophageal malignancy invade these structures, an R0 curative resection may not be technically feasible.

The complex submucosal lymphatic network of the esophagus also renders it prone to widespread lymphatic metastases. For example, tumors that invade the submucosa have a greater than 20% incidence of lymph node metastasis, whereas tumors that invade the deeper layers of the submucosa can exhibit a 45% incidence of lymphatic metastases.[5,6] Early submucosal involvement by cancer can render the patient prone to widespread and distant lymphatic metastasis, even in the absence of negative lymph nodes located near or adjacent to the primary tumor, a process referred to as "skip" metastasis. Thus, in cases of suspicious nodal involvement, and/or in cases of transmural tumor extension (ie, most of T2 and all of T3 and T4 lesions), neoadjuvant induction therapy is commonly used before operation.

Given the aforementioned challenges regarding the gross and lymphatic anatomy of the esophagus, the particular technique of esophagectomy and extent of resection is often a matter of debate. Regardless of the esophagectomy technique, the primary goal of this operation when performed for carcinoma is an *R0 resection*. As long as the surgeon can achieve this goal, the technique of resection can theoretically be left to the surgeon's decision; although, this does in fact remain controversial.

ANASTOMOTIC TECHNIQUES

When performing the esophageal anastomosis, several factors are important to consider. One of these factors includes the location of the anastomosis, to include either an intrathoracic or cervical location. Also, the choice of the esophageal replacement conduit can be dependent on the particular clinical scenario. The stomach is the most commonly used conduit for esophageal reconstruction. However, the esophageal surgeon may encounter a scenario where the stomach cannot be used as a conduit, such as the situation in which a history of prior gastric surgery prohibits the use of the stomach. When this is the case, reconstruction options can include the use of a colonic interposition reconstruction, or a jejunal interposition graft. An additional important factor to consider with regard to the esophageal anastomosis involves the technical aspect involved in the creation of the anastomosis, regardless of the conduit choice. These so-called technical aspects are discussed in this text and include the total mechanical technique, the semimechanical technique, and the fully hand-sewn technique. Also, the orientation of the anastomosis is included in this aspect and includes the end-to-end, end-to-side, and side-to-side anastomosis (**Table 1**).

CERVICAL ANASTOMOTIC TECHNIQUES

Cervical anastomoses, as performed in the transhiatal and 3-field (McKeown) approaches, are carried out via 2 main techniques: the semimechanical technique as described by Dr Orringer and colleagues,[7] which involves a combination of a linear cutting stapler and hand sewing to complete the anastomosis in the neck; and the total mechanical technique described by Dr Landreneau and colleagues.[8]

Semimechanical Cervical Anastomosis

A left-sided neck incision is made anterior to the sternocleidomastoid muscle, the omohyoid muscle is divided, the carotid sheath is identified and retracted laterally, and the larynx and thyroid cartilage is retracted medially. The dissection is continued posteriorly to the prevertebral fascia; the esophagus is identified, encircled bluntly taking care to identify and protect the left recurrent laryngeal nerve, and brought up into the field. Next, blunt dissection is carried as far down as possible into the mediastinum, ideally to the carinal level. The tubularized gastric conduit is mobilized and passed via the hiatus through the mediastinum and delivered via the left neck incision. The proximal esophagus is divided with an endovascular gastrointestinal anastomosis (endo GIA) linear cutting stapler.

A side-to-side esophagogastrostomy is then created as described by Orringer and colleagues.[7] An approximately 1.5-cm gastrotomy is made a few centimeters proximal to the edge of the conduit. While performing this gastrotomy, it is important to keep in mind how much proximal esophagus is available to perform the anastomosis and the size of the staple cartridge, as these factors may require the need to alter the location of the gastrotomy. The proximal esophagus is then grasped with atraumatic forceps and the staple line is cut in an oblique fashion in such a way that the anterior portion is slightly longer than the posterior portion, as this serves to shape the anastomosis. This amputated staple line is sent to pathology as the proximal margin (**Fig. 1**).

The gastric conduit is placed over the prevertebral fascia and the esophageal stump is placed over the tip of gastric conduit anteriorly. Subsequently, 2 full-thickness stay sutures using 4 to 0 Vicryl, are placed that facilitate traction in preparation for the creation of the anastomosis. First, a stay suture is placed at the anterior portion of the esophagus, whereas the second is placed through the posterior edge of the esophagus and then through the superior edge of the gastrotomy. The endo GIA stapler is then positioned with the cartridge placed within the esophagus and the anvil portion placed within the gastric conduit (see **Fig. 1**). The aforementioned traction sutures are used to help position the stapler before the firing. It is important to ensure that the posterior wall

Table 1		
The esophageal anastomosis type with regard to location and orientation		
Types of anastomosis	**Intrathoracic**	**Cervical**
Hand-sewn anastomosis	End-to-end	End-to-end
Semimechanical anastomosis	End-to-side	End-to-end
Total mechanical anastomosis	End-to-side	End-to-side

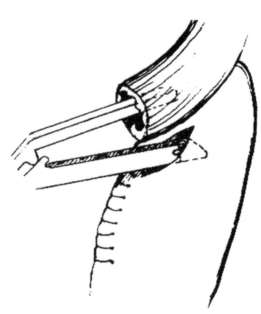

Fig. 1. Creation of the posterolateral aspect of the esophagogastric anastomosis. (*From* Santos RS, Raftopoulos Y, Singh D, DeHoyos A, Fernando HC, Keenan RJ, Luketich JD, Landreneau RJ: Utility of total mechanical stapled cervical esophagogastric anastomosis after esophagectomy: A comparison to conventional anastomotic techniques. Surgery. 2004;136(4):917-925, with permission.)

of the esophagus aligns to the anterior wall of the stomach. Once proper stapler positioning is confirmed, the stapler is then fired while providing traction on the previously placed sutures. This creates the posterior portion of the esophagogastric anastomosis.

Following firing of the stapler, a nasogastric tube is passed under direct vision into the gastric conduit. Next, the anterior portion of the anastomosis is performed via a 2-layered hand-sewn technique. A running, full-thickness suture line is created by running two 4 to 0 polydioxanone (PDS) sutures from the corners of both sides and having them meet in the middle and tied (**Fig. 2**). During this portion, it is extremely important to ensure mucosal apposition. Following this layer, interrupted 4 to 0 PDS sutures are then placed in Lembert fashion to complete the second layer of the anterior hand-sewn portion of the anastomosis. The anastomosis is usually located 19 to 20 cm from incisors.

Before closure, a peri-anastomotic drain is left in situ, either via a separate stab incision or within the left cervical incision.

Totally Mechanical Cervical Anastomosis

The total mechanical cervical anastomotic technique resembles the semimechanical technique described previously with some exceptions. Instead of the esophagus lying on the anterior surface of the gastric conduit, both the esophagus and gastric conduit are rolled up to create a side-by-side anastomosis. The gastrostomy is performed at the apex of the gastric conduit rather than anterior surface. A 30-mm or 45-mm endo-stapler is used to staple the posterior wall of the esophageal stump to the greater curvature of the gastric conduit. Subsequently, Allis clamps are placed strategically to orient and line up the tissue margins. This can be accomplished by placing separate Allis clamps on the lateral edges of the posterior staple line and one Allis clamp placed

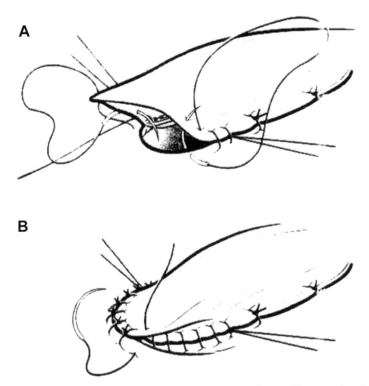

Fig. 2. Two-layer suturing approach: a running inner layer of monofilament absorbable suture (A) and an outer interrupted layer that incorporates the anterior wall of the upper esophagus (B). (From Santos RS, Raftopoulos Y, Singh D, DeHoyos A, Fernando HC, Keenan RJ, Luketich JD, Landreneau RJ: Utility of total mechanical stapled cervical esophagogastric anastomosis after esophagectomy: A comparison to conventional anastomotic techniques. Surgery. 2004;136(4):917-925, with permission.)

on the anterior aspect of the esophagus and stomach.[8] Before firing the stapler to complete the anterior aspect of the anastomosis, it is important to ensure that the submucosa and mucosa are within the staple line of the anterior portion of the anastomosis. Either an endo-stapler or a TA stapler is used to complete the anastomosis (**Fig. 3**).

Following completion of the anastomosis, a peri-anastomotic drain is placed via a separate cervical stab incision.

Landreneau and colleagues found that the total mechanical anastomosis decreased the operative time, as well as the rate of postoperative strictures requiring dilation. Thus, it is argued that the total mechanical anastomosis creates a wider anastomosis when compared to the hand-sewn techniques.[8]

MINIMALLY INVASIVE THORACIC ANASTOMOTIC TECHNIQUES

In United States, almost 50% of esophagectomies are performed via the Ivor Lewis approach with an intrathoracic anastomosis.[9] The basic principles of the intrathoracic anastomosis include a complete mobilization of the esophagus superior to azygous level, enough conduit length to perform a tension-free anastomosis with optional reinforcement with omentum, and avoidance of injury to structures such as the mainstem

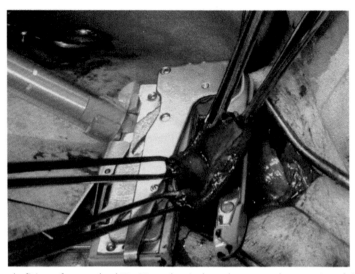

Fig. 3. Single firing of a standard TA-60 mechanical stapler across the margins of the esophagus and stomach. (*From* Santos RS, Raftopoulos Y, Singh D, DeHoyos A, Fernando HC, Keenan RJ, Luketich JD, Landreneau RJ: Utility of total mechanical stapled cervical esophagogastric anastomosis after esophagectomy: A comparison to conventional anastomotic techniques. Surgery. 2004;136(4):917-925, with permission.)

bronchi, azygous vein, aorta, and thoracic duct during creation of the anastomosis. Several techniques of minimally invasive intrathoracic anastomosis have been described using both video-assisted minimally invasive esophagectomy (MIE) and robotic-assisted minimally invasive esophagectomy (RAMIE) approaches.

There is literature to support that the performance of an intrathoracic anastomosis carries a reduction in the risk of an anastomotic leak when compared with a cervical anastomosis. In particular, an analysis of the Society of Thoracic Surgeons database published in 2013 showed a statistically significant reduction in risk in favor of an intrathoracic anastomosis (9.3% vs 12.3%), although the analysis also found that there was no significant difference in mortality associated with an anastomotic leak between the cervical versus the thoracic anastomotic technique.[10]

Both the MIE and RAMIE are shown to have comparable outcomes with the open approach. The studies have shown that both the MIE and RAMIE approaches are non-inferior to open approaches regarding long-term survival in patients with esophageal carcinoma with a significantly higher lymph node harvest when compared with open esophagectomy.[11]

When comparing the MIE approach to the RAMIE, the latter has not been proven to be superior to the MIE approach.[12,13]

The common approaches of thoracoscopic or robotic intrathoracic anastomosis creation are listed as follows:

- Hand-sewn anastomosis
- Completely mechanical anastomosis
  - Traditional end-to-end anastomosis (EEA) circular stapler
  - EEA OrVil device (Medtronic)
- Semimechanical anastomosis

Circular Stapler/End-to-End Anastomosis Purse-String Technique

After the completion of esophageal mobilization, the esophagus is cut either using an endoscopic or robotic monopolar scissors. The proximal part of the anastomosis requires the placement of the anvil in the esophageal stump and placement of a running baseball purse-string suture. Most investigators will place the anvil in the esophageal stump first followed by placing the purse-string suture in MIE; however, during a RAMIE, the purse-string suture is placed first followed by insertion of the anvil in the esophageal stump. It is important to ensure that the purse-string suture incorporates the mucosa and the esophageal wall. With the anvil in place, this purse-string suture is then tied down and secured. If this purse-sting suture is not deemed to be adequately tight around the anvil, a second purse string can then be placed outside of the original purse string to secure the esophagus tightly around the anvil (**Fig. 4**). This outer edge of the esophagus must be flat after securing the purse string and before docking it to the handle side of the EEA stapler to ensure that the overlying tissue is not excessively thick and thus lead to a better purchase of tissue with the stapler itself.[14] The most frequent circular stapler size used for anastomosis is 28 mm followed by 25 mm.

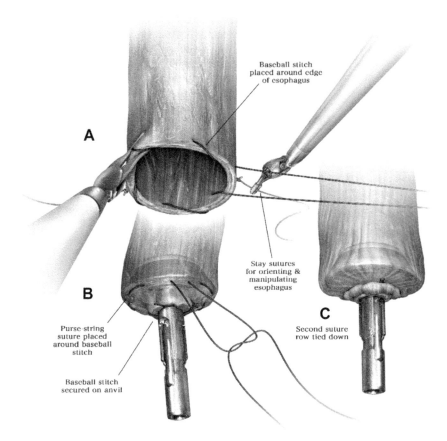

Fig. 4. The purse-string EEA technique. (*From* Caso R, Wee JO: Esophagogastric Anastomotic Techniques for Minimally Invasive and Robotic Ivor Lewis Operations. Operative Techniques in Thoracic and Cardiovascular Surgery 25: 105-123, 2020, with permission.)

Higher sizes are used in cases of a severely dilated esophagus, as is often the case in patients with end-stage achalasia.

The handle of the EEA stapler is introduced by enlarging the posterior port site. The gastric conduit is then brought up and oriented to ensure that it is not twisted and will lie tension-free within the thoracic cavity. Next, the proximal portion of the gastric conduit is opened along the staple line and the handle of the EEA stapler is placed within the gastric conduit. The spike of the EEA handle is then placed through the gastric wall along the greater curvature. The spike is then docked under direct thoracoscopic vision with manipulation by the surgeon to connect it to the anvil. After docking, the surgeon must be sure that there is minimal to no redundancy of the conduit before firing the stapler. The anvil is then inspected for the 2 "donuts" of esophageal tissue that indicate a successful staple firing. These 2 donuts are then sent off the field to pathology as the "final proximal margin." Following successful completion of the anastomosis, the open end of the gastric conduit from which the handle was placed is resected with an endo-stapler and sent off the field as the "final distal margin" (**Fig. 5**).

After completing the gastric resection, the surgeon may choose to reinforce and/or buttress the anastomosis staple line with fatty tissue, or with a portion of omentum if harvested during the abdominal portion of the operation. Once compete, appropriate drains are placed: our practice is to place a 28-Fr chest tube directed to the apex of the right hemithorax, as well as a peri-anastomotic 10-Fr flat Jackson Pratt drain.

The robotic-assisted EEA purse-string technique is performed in a similar fashion to the thoracoscopic EEA purse-string technique with the circular stapler. Similarly, the esophagus is transected sharply using the robotic scissors. The surgeon may choose to place separate stay sutures on the lateral and medial edges of the transected esophagus to help orient and align it with the gastric conduit before completing the anastomosis.

Circular Stapler Using OrVil (Transoral) End-to-End Anastomosis Stapler

This technique is almost similar to the circular stapler/EEA purse-string technique except that the anvil of EEA stapler is introduced through the mouth, mounted on a

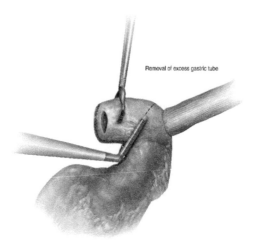

Fig. 5. Excising the excess stomach via the use of a linear cutting stapler. The resected stomach serves as the "final distal margin." (*From* Tsai WS, Levy RM, Luketich JD: Technique of Minimally Invasive Ivor Lewis Esophagectomy. Operative Techniques in Thoracic and Cardiovascular Surgery: A Comparative Atlas 14: 176-192, 2009, with permission.)

nasogastric tube, and passed into the esophageal stump. This technique is regarded to perhaps be slightly faster than use of standard EEA stapler. The limitation with this technique is that largest size available is 25 mm.[15] The esophagus is mobilized in the usual fashion and stapled just above the azygous vein either using a manual stapler or robotic stapler. In our practice, the transection of the esophagus is few centimeters above the azygous vein, which is consistently 23 to 24 cm from the incisor teeth. The anvil portion of the OrVil (Medtronic, Minneapolis, MN) comes already attached via suture to a nasogastric tube in a separate pack than the DST EEA 25-mm stapler. The anvil is passed through the mouth. As the nasogastric tube is passed transorally, usually by an anesthesia colleague, it is important to ensure that the metal anvil is guided through the patient's oropharynx so it does not cause injury to this area or become entangled around the endotracheal tube. Once the tip of the nasogastric tube is visualized against the blind pouch of esophageal stump, a hole is created in the middle of the stump just below the staple line, either using hot endo-shear during MIE or robotic electrocautery during RAMIE, to allow for the extrusion of the tip of nasogastric tube. The bedside assistant in RAMIE, or the surgeon during MIE, then grasps the nasogastric tube and pulls it out while the anesthesiologist introduces the anvil attached to the other end of the nasogastric tube in the patient's mouth and facilitates its passage to avoid cervical esophageal injury. The sutures that attach the nasogastric tube to the anvil are then cut and the nasogastric tube is subsequently removed, and the anvil is situated similar to the EEA/purse-string technique described previously (**Fig. 6**). At this time, a purse-string suture using a "0" silk is placed around the base of the anvil to further secure it within the esophagus. The handle of the EEA stapler is then passed via the postero-inferior port after slightly enlarging this

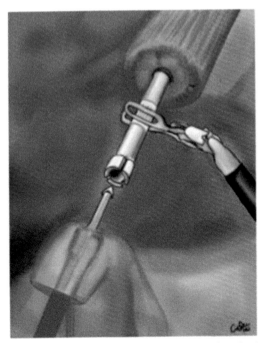

Fig. 6. Anastomosis using an EEA stapler. (*From* Musgrove et al. Robotic assisted minimally invasive esophagectomy: Ivor-Lewis approach. Shanghai Chest 2020.)

incision.[16] The anastomosis is then performed using the previously described EEA/purse-string technique.

Intrathoracic anastomosis using linear stapler

The anastomotic technique that uses the linear stapler is thought to create a wider anastomosis and thus reduces the incidence of postoperative anastomotic strictures, especially when compared with hand-sewn techniques.[17] A slightly longer gastric conduit is needed in this technique. The esophagus is transected above the level of azygous vein using the endo-shear robotic scissors. The gastric conduit is placed under the esophageal stump (similar to the technique of Orringer and colleagues[7] mentioned in the neck anastomosis section). Two stay sutures are placed on each side to anchor the esophageal stump to gastric conduit. A gastrotomy is created on the anterior wall of the gastric conduit so that it may accept the cartridge portion of the linear stapler. After the stapler is in place, it is fired so that a side-to-side esophagogastrostomy is created. After firing and subsequent removal of the linear stapler, the defect in the anastomosis from where access for the stapler was provided is sutured with thoracoscopic or robotic suturing instruments in 2 layers (**Fig. 7**). The linear stapler used can be manual or robotic. This intrathoracic technique mimics the previously described cervical anastomosis technique of Orringer and colleagues.[7] During RAMIE, the authors use two 3 to 0 *V-Loc* sutures (Medtronic) to close the anterior defect after the removal of the stapler. Each suture is started at the end, meeting in the middle.

Hand Sewn

A hand-sewn end-to-end or end-to-side esophagogastric anastomosis can be accomplished thoracoscopically or robotically as well. For this technique, the transected esophagus is sewn at its posterior wall to the gastrotomy created on the greater curvature of the gastric conduit with thoracoscopic suturing instruments/graspers using seromuscular suture bites in interrupted fashion with PDS sutures. It should also be noted that the posterior anastomosis may be sutured in a running fashion with a self-locking suture such as a *V-Loc* (Medtronic) or *Stratafix* (Ethicon, Somerville, NJ). This anastomosis is completed in an end-to-side fashion (**Fig. 8**). The double-armed suture begins in the "middle" of the posterior aspect of the anastomosis and is carried out toward both "ends" of the anastomosis. It is paramount to achieve mucosal-to-

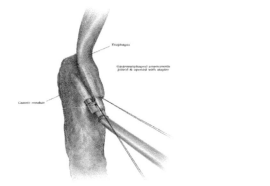
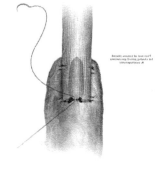

Fig. 7. The linear staple anastomosis. (*From* Caso R, Wee JO: Esophagogastric Anastomotic Techniques for Minimally Invasive and Robotic Ivor Lewis Operations. Operative Techniques in Thoracic and Cardiovascular Surgery 25: 105-123, 2020, with permission.)

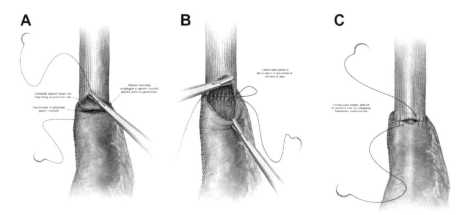

Fig. 8. The thoracoscopic hand-sewn technique. (*From* Caso R, Wee JO: Esophagogastric Anastomotic Techniques for Minimally Invasive and Robotic Ivor Lewis Operations. Operative Techniques in Thoracic and Cardiovascular Surgery 25: 105-123, 2020, with permission.)

mucosal apposition when performing a hand-sewn anastomotic technique. To ensure this, the surgeon may elect to place a Connell stich, which is used to invert the wall of the esophagus and stomach by passing the suture first through the outside of the intestinal wall and then passing it back through the ipsilateral lumen and then repeating this pattern on the contralateral side of the anastomosis, at each end of the posterior suture line, as this inverts the suture line to further ensure apposition of the mucosae. Following completion of the posterior suture line, a nasogastric tube is passed under direct vision. The anterior aspect of the anastomosis is then completed with a running suture technique.

Robotic-Assisted Hand-Sewn Technique

In the robotic-assisted hand-sewn technique, the robotic platform (Intuitive, Sunnyvale, CA) provides more freedom of movement, as it allows for pitch, yaw, and roll in regard to the suturing of the anastomosis, as well as superior visualization when compared with the thoracoscopic technique. In this robotic-assisted technique, a 2-layered or a single-layer anastomosis is performed with the use of the robotic suturing instruments.

The anastomosis is carried out by first determining a location on the gastric conduit at least 3 cm inferior from the apex of the gastric conduit. This location is where the gastrotomy is made for the subsequent anastomosis. While performing this step, it is important to create the gastrotomy as distant as possible from the staple line on the lesser curvature. The posterior layer is sutured first and is performed by placing interrupted 3 to 0 permanent suture (ie, silk) to approximate the posterior muscular layer of the esophagus to the seromuscular layer of the gastric conduit. Following the creation of this posterior suture line, the inner layer of the anastomosis is performed. This is carried out using a 3 to 0 PDS suture in running fashion. This suture line begins on the medial portion of the anastomosis. Once the posterior inner running layer is completed, a 3 to 0 PDS is began on the lateral inner portion of the anastomosis and is run anteriorly to meet the suture that was brought out from the medial aspect of the anastomosis.[15] The anterior outer/second layer is then performed in an interrupted fashion using a 3 to 0 permanent suture. It should also be noted that some surgeons may elect to perform this anastomosis using a single layer, as opposed to a 2-layer anastomosis. This can be performed with any monofilament suture. An auto-locking suture (ie, Stratafix or V-Loc) also can be used, as it may offer the advantage of not having to maintain tension on the suture while suturing due to its barbs.

Although the robotic-assisted approach offers many advantages to the performance of an esophagogastric anastomosis in the chest, there are some disadvantages associated with this technique. These include the steep learning curve inherent to this technique, the longer operative time necessary to successfully complete this technique, and the costs of the robot. However, despite these disadvantages, the advantages that the robot provides will likely continue to outweigh these shortcomings, especially as experience grows over time and surgeons become more adept and experienced with this approach.

ADDITIONAL AREAS OF DISCUSSION
Coverage of the Anastomosis with Omentum

After completion of the esophagogastric anastomosis, many surgeons buttress the anastomosis with autologous tissue, namely the omentum. It is our practice to harvest a vascularized portion of the greater omentum when preparing the conduit within the abdomen. The omental flap is then passed into the chest or neck with the conduit and is clipped with a clipping device or sutured adjacent to the staple line so that it covers the actual anastomosis. A retrospective review from MD Anderson Cancer Center of more than 600 patients, where 35% of these patients underwent an intrathoracic anastomosis buttressed by omentum, showed a statistically significant decrease in the anastomotic leak rate when the intrathoracic anastomosis is reinforced by a pedicled tongue of omentum compared with anastomoses that were not buttressed by omentum.[18] Thus, the utilization of a pedicled omental flap to reinforce the esophageal anastomosis may serve a significant benefit in that it may decrease the risk of a clinically significant anastomotic leak.

Anastomotic Strictures

A retrospective review by Price and colleagues[19] of 525 patients undergoing esophagectomy demonstrated that there were no significant differences in the incidence of anastomotic stricture with regard to the anastomotic technique when the anastomosis was performed in the neck. However, this review did identify a statistically significant decrease in the incidence of anastomotic stricture with the linear stapled technique compared with the hand-sewn or circular technique when the anastomosis was performed in the chest.[19] A retrospective review or 293 patients by Xu and colleagues[20] also demonstrated a decrease in anastomotic stricture rate with the linear stapled technique when compared with the hand-sewn and circular stapled techniques.

Simulation Training in Construction of the Esophagogastric Anastomosis

As the creation of the intrathoracic esophageal anastomosis via minimally invasive techniques becomes more prevalent and its use widespread, it is well-known that this operation is complex and is associated with a steep learning curve. There have been publications demonstrating the benefit of simulation training with regard to practice of the creation of the intrathoracic esophagogastric anastomosis via the minimally invasive technique via a simulated model.[21] Thus, the utilization of simulation models may revolutionize the way in which these complex techniques are taught and enable the current generation of surgical trainees to become facile with these anastomotic techniques before actually performing them within the operating room on a patient.

SUMMARY

As the techniques of esophagectomy, postoperative care, and neoadjuvant therapies continue to evolve, it is paramount for the esophageal surgeon to possess multiple anastomotic techniques within their armamentarium. As each case is complex and different, depending on the location of the tumor, size of the tumor, and so forth, a particular anastomotic technique may be better suited for a particular case when compared with another technique. Each anastomosis described has its own particular advantages and disadvantages. Fortunately, several techniques for the esophagogastric anastomosis exist and it is up to the surgeon to become facile and adept with these multiple anastomotic techniques.

CLINICS CARE POINTS

- The techniques of esophagectomy continue to evolve. The advent of minimally invasive techniques, such as the totally laparoscopic and thoracoscopic, as well as the RAMIE, have transformed the landscape with regard to this operation.
- Several techniques exist to create the esophagogastric anastomosis.
- The anastomosis can be created via a total mechanical stapled approach, a fully hand-sewn approach, or a combination of the two: the semimechanical approach
- Although there are a variety of techniques for the esophagogastric anastomosis, several basic principles apply regardless of the technique chosen:
  ○ The anastomosis must be created so that it is free of tension with adequate blood supply.
  ○ The location of the tumor dictates the location of the anastomosis (ie, a proximal cancer may necessitate a cervical anastomosis).
  ○ The esophageal surgeon must be facile and adept at various techniques in creating the esophagogastric anastomosis.

DISCLOSURE

The authors have no financial disclosures with regard to this article.

REFERENCES

1. Howlader NNA, Krapcho M, Miller D, et al. SEER Cancer Statistics Review. In. Based on November 2018 SEER data submission. National Cancer Institute. Bethesda, MD. Available at: https://seer.cancer.gov/%20csr/1975_2016/.
2. Cunningham D, Allum WH, Stenning SP, et al. Perioperative chemotherapy versus surgery alone for resectable gastro-esophageal cancer. N Engl J Med 2006;355: 11–20.
3. Al-Batran S-E, Homann N, Pauligk C, et al. Perioperative chemotherapy with fluorouracil plus leucovorin, oxaliplatin, and docetaxel versus fluorouracil or capecitabine plus cisplatin and epirubicin for locally advanced, resectable gastric or gastro-oesophageal junction adenocarcinoma (FLOT4): a randomised, phase 2/3 trial. Lancet 2019;393:1948–57.
4. Lerut T, Moons J, Coosemans W, et al. Multidisciplinary treatment of advanced cancer of the esophagus and gastroesophageal junction: a European center's approach. Surg Oncol Clin N Am 2008;17:485–502, vii–viii.
5. Leers JM, DeMeester SR, Oezcelik A, et al. The prevalence of lymph node metastases in patients with T1 esophageal adenocarcinoma: a retrospective review of esophagectomy specimens. Ann Surg 2011;253(2):271–8.

6. Raja S, Rice TW, Goldblum JR, et al. Esophageal submucosa: the watershed for esophageal cancer. J Thorac Cardiovasc Surg 2011;142:1403–11.
7. Orringer MB, Marshall B, Iannettoni MD. Eliminating the cervical esophagogastric anastomotic leak with a side-to-side stapled anastomosis. J Thorac Cardiovasc Surg 2000;119:277–88.
8. Santos RS, Raftopoulos Y, Singh D, et al. Utility of total mechanical stapled cervical esophagogastric anastomosis after esophagectomy: a comparison to conventional anastomotic techniques. Surgery 2004;136(4):917–25.
9. Pennathur A, Awais O, Luketich JD. Technique of minimally invasive Ivor Lewis esophagectomy. Ann Thorac Surg 2010;89(6):S2159–62.
10. Kassis ES, Kosinski AS, Ross P, et al. Predictors of anastomotic leak after esophagectomy: an analysis of the Society of Thoracic Surgeons General Thoracic Surgical Database. Ann Thorac Surg 2013;96(6):1919–26.
11. Espinoza-Mercado F, Imai TA, Borgella JD, et al. Does the approach matter? Comparing survival in robotic, minimally invasive, and open esophagectomies. Ann Thorac Surg 2019;107:378–85.
12. Wei B, D'Amico TA. Thoracoscopic versus robotic approaches: advantages and disadvantages. Thorac Surg Clin 2014;24:177–88, vi.
13. Harbison GJ, Vossler JD, Yim NH, et al. Outcomes of robotic versus non-robotic minimally-invasive esophagectomy for esophageal cancer: An American College of Surgeons NSQIP database analysis. Am J Surg 2019;218:1223–8.
14. Naffouje SA, Salloum RH, Khalaf Z, et al. Outcomes of open versus minimally invasive Ivor-Lewis esophagectomy for cancer: a propensity-score matched analysis of NSQIP database. Ann Surg Oncol 2019;26:2001–10.
15. Caso R, Wee JO. Esophagogastric anastomotic techniques for minimally invasive and robotic ivor lewis operations. Oper Tech Thorac Cardiovasc Surg 2020;25: 105–23.
16. Musgrove K, Spear CR, Kakuturu J, et al. Robotic assisted minimally invasive esophagectomy: Ivor-Lewis approach. Shanghai Chest 2020.
17. Ercan S, Rice TW, Murthy SC, et al. Does esophagogastric anastomotic technique influence the outcome of patients with esophageal cancer? J Thorac Cardiovasc Surg 2005;129:623–31.
18. Sepesi B, Swisher SG, Walsh GL, et al. Omental reinforcement of the thoracic esophagogastric anastomosis: An analysis of leak and reintervention rates in patients undergoing planned and salvage esophagectomy. J Thorac Cardiovasc Surg 2012;144:1146–51.
19. Price TN, Nichols FC, Harmsen WS, et al. A comprehensive review of anastomotic technique in 432 esophagectomies. Ann Thorac Surg 2013;95:1154–61.
20. Xu QR, Wang KN, Wang WP, et al. Linear stapled esophagogastrostomy is more effective than hand-sewn or circular stapler in prevention of anastomotic stricture: a comparative clinical study. J Gastrointest Surg 2011;15(6):915–21.
21. Fabian T, Glotzer OS, Bakhos CT. Construct validation: simulation of thoracoscopic intrathoracic anastomosis. JSLS 2015;19(2). e2015.00001.

Management of Postoperative Complications After Esophageal Resection

Thomas Fabian, MD

KEYWORDS

- Esophagectomy complications • Esophageal anastomotic leak
- Morbidity following esophagectomy • Pneumonia following esophagectomy

KEY POINTS

- Complications following esophagectomy are common.
- Avoidance of complications through technical improvements remain paramount.
- Mitigation of complications is critical to minimize morbidity and mortality.

 Video content accompanies this article at http://www.surgical.theclinics.com.

INTRODUCTION

According to the Surveillance, Epidemiology, and End Results Program,[1] in 2019, the most common esophageal malignancy was esophageal adenocarcinoma followed by squamous cell carcinoma. Stage at the time of diagnosis was distant (IV) in 40%, regional in 32%, localized in 18%, and unknown in 10%. Treatment in the United States consists of chemotherapy in 61.7% of patients, followed by radiotherapy in 55.4% of patients, followed by surgery.[2] Only 26.6% of all esophageal cancers underwent surgical resection, although it was more common in adenocarcinoma (32.9%) than in squamous cell carcinoma (15.9%).

Newer surgical techniques have reduced complications and mortality following esophagectomy,[3–5] but they nevertheless remain high. In a multi-institutional phase 2 trial, Luketich and colleagues[3] reported that 52 (49.5%) of 104 patients undergoing esophagectomy had Grade 3 or Grade 4 complications within 30 days of surgery. We found similar results within our own group, with 59% of our patients suffering complications.[5] Although most of those complications were minor, 23% of our patients suffered major complications.

Section of Thoracic Surgery, Albany Medical College, Third Floor, 50 New Scotland Avenue, Albany, NY 12159, USA
E-mail address: Fabiant@amc.edu

Surg Clin N Am 101 (2021) 525–539
https://doi.org/10.1016/j.suc.2021.03.013
surgical.theclinics.com
0039-6109/21/© 2021 Elsevier Inc. All rights reserved.

Data regarding complications are frequently inconsistent and therefore difficult to compare. In 2015, Low and colleagues[6] were the lead investigators for the Esophagectomy Complications Consensus Group (ECCG). This group established standardized criteria based on a platform of 9 systems. These criteria included pulmonary, cardiac, gastrointestinal, urologic, thromboembolic, neurologic/psychiatric, infection, wound/diaphragm, and others (chyle leak). They further defined and staged the severity of anastomotic leaks, conduit necrosis, chyle leak, and vocal cord injury. The ECCG analyzed data from 14 countries and 24 institutions worldwide.[7] The most common complications reported were pneumonia (14.6%), arrythmia (14.5%), anastomotic leak (11.4%), chylothorax (4.7%), recurrent laryngeal nerve palsy (RNLP) (4.2%), and conduit necrosis (1.3%) **(Table 1)**. These data were confirmed by the work of many others including Ozawa and colleagues[8] who reported the incidence of pneumonia, arrhythmia, anastomotic leak, and RNLP all to be approximately 10% in each. We found similar outcomes in our own published series.[5] Our incidence of pneumonia was 14%, atrial fibrillation 15%, anastomotic leak 9%, RNLP 5%, chylothorax 3%, and gastric tip necrosis 1.5%. In that study, published in 2006, we found no difference in overall occurrence of complications between minimally invasive esophagectomy (MIE) and open esophagectomy (OE). In comparing the 2 techniques, overall complications occurred in 59% in the MIE group and 72% in the OE group, and major complications occurred in 23% and 30%, respectively, although the risk of respiratory failure requiring ventilation was less in the MIE group (5%) versus the OE group (23%) with $P = .002$.

These publications highlight short-term complications; however, long-term complications such as dysphagia, stricture, delayed gastric emptying, bile reflux, aspiration, and post-esophagectomy hiatal hernias are significant as well.

To analyze long-term quality-of-life issues, Scarpa and colleagues[9] published a meta-analysis on health-related quality of life (HRQL) after esophagectomy. They reported that compared with normal individuals, patients post-esophagectomy complained of worsened fatigue, dyspnea, and diarrhea 6 months after esophagectomy. In contrast, emotional function had significantly improved after 6 months. In conclusion, short-term and long-term HRQL is deeply affected after esophagectomy

Table 1 Esophagectomy complications consensus group	
Complication	**Incidence, %**
Pneumonia	14.6
Arrythmia	14.5
Anastomotic leak	11.4
Chylothorax	4.7
Recurrent laryngeal nerve palsy	4.2
Conduit necrosis	1.3
Readmission rates	11.2
Mortality rate	
30 day	2.4
90 day	4.5
Total	59

Data from Low, D.E., et al., Benchmarking Complications Associated with Esophagectomy. Ann Surg 2019;269(2):291-8.

for cancer. The investigators concluded that impairment of physical function may be a long-term consequence of esophagectomy involving either the respiratory system or the alimentary tract.

Surgical resection of the esophagus remains a mainstay of treatment. Surgical excision for early-stage and localized tumors is frequently curative, although there are cures with concurrent chemoradiation as was discussed in an earlier article in this issue. Curative outcomes are limited. In RTOG 85 to 01, Cooper and colleagues[10] reported survival with chemoradiation of 26% at 5 years and overall survival of 14%. To improve survival of this cancer, it seems paramount to offer successful surgery to a larger number of resectable patients. Dubecz and colleagues[11] analyzed multiple databases to review care of 23,000 patients with esophageal cancer and reported that only 44% of subjects with potentially resectable disease underwent surgery.

It stands to reason that if 56% of the patients are not offered curative treatment, overall survival would remain low. In 2019, the 5-year survival of patients with esophageal cancer in the United States was only 19.9%.[1] This is in part due to the generalized perception that esophageal cancer and its treatments are morbid, and that the malignancy is rarely cured. As a result, many physicians take a nihilistic approach to these malignancies. In practice, we frequently talk to patients and their families regarding the role of surgery. We find that in many of these patients it has been suggested to them that surgery is not necessary, not worth it, or even that it should be avoided in persistent disease. This negative perception results in undertreatment of many cancers, which in turn results in worse overall outcomes. Dubecz and colleagues[11] also demonstrated geography and access to care as an important issue. Although only 44% of surgical candidates underwent surgical resection in the State of New York, the number was much higher at certain centers. Of patients who underwent treatment at a specialized care center, 64% underwent esophagectomy as part of their treatment.

To optimize care for esophageal cancer, we need to offer patients a surgical resection that minimizes and mitigates complications when they inevitably occur. This article attempts to review contemporary data on common complications and their management in the hope of assisting the reader in the accomplishment of that goal.

ANASTOMOTIC LEAKS

Anastomotic leaks following esophagectomy are not uncommon, occurring in 11.4% of esophagectomies in the ECCG.[6] Anastomotic leaks occur more frequently in the neck than in the chest. They can be difficult to solve and can ultimately be life threatening. Techniques to minimize this complication are important. Optimizing blood supply with a wider conduit and creating the anastomosis in the chest are widely considered beneficial. In a contemporary series of MIE, Bizekis and colleagues,[4] from the University of Pittsburgh, described modifying their minimally invasive technique to Ivor Lewis esophagectomy with an intrathoracic anastomotic leak rate of only 6%.

When comparing outcomes in patients with anastomotic leaks, it is important to define those leaks. The ECCG[6] and the Surgical Infection Study Group (SISS)[12] both defined and graded anastomotic leaks (**Table 2**). Although similar, the SISS group included clinical behavior of the patient. The SISS group also had a Grade 4, which is gastric necrosis leading to leak or sepsis. With regard to treatment, in both groups, small anastomotic leaks are either observed or frequently left with a nasogastric tube (NGT) as management. Most of these leaks will heal without intervention provided there is no distal obstruction, but specific recommendations are lacking.

Table 2
Definitions of anastomotic leaks

Esophagectomy Complications Consensus Group[6]	Surgical Infection Study Group[12]
• Type I: Local defect requiring no change in therapy or treated medically • Type II: Localized defect requiring interventional but not surgical therapy • Type III: Localized defect requiring surgical therapy.	• Grade 1 (radiologically or endoscopically detected): without clinical signs • Grade 2 (minor clinical): local inflammation • Grade 3 (major clinical): severe disruption with sepsis • Grade 4 (conduit necrosis): confirmed by endoscopy.

From Low, D.E., et al., International Consensus on Standardization of Data Collection for Complications Associated With Esophagectomy: Esophagectomy Complications Consensus Group (ECCG). Ann Surg, 2015. 262(2): p. 286-94; and Peel, A.L. and E.W. Taylor, Proposed definitions for the audit of postoperative infection: a discussion paper. Surgical Infection Study Group. Ann R Coll Surg Engl, 1991. 73(6): p. 385-8.

Verstegen and colleagues[13] attempted to review the literature and provided management recommendations from 19 retrospective studies. Citing poor methodology in those studies and discrepancies in descriptions of patients, they concluded there was no evidence supporting a specific treatment for anastomotic leaks and that management should be customized for each situation. In that review, mortality occurred in 8% of patients with cervical anastomotic leak.

When discussing management of anastomotic leaks, considerations should include location, size of leak, time since surgery, emptying of the conduit, and the patient's clinical status and stability. Also relevant is how the leak was discovered. Although some surgeons choose not to evaluate their anastomosis postoperatively, some do so with an esophagram and others with endoscopy. These data support all 3 approaches. When a leak is identified, all patients should undergo endoscopic evaluation. Gastric tip necrosis must be excluded, and this can be done only with endoscopy. At the time of endoscopy, the pylorus should be evaluated and dilated if need be, and any mediastinal contamination with contrast should be cleaned. It is at this time the surgeon should determine what initial management approach to take.

Anastomoses created in the neck do not always remain in the neck, and this is an important consideration. Cervical anastomotic leaks that are not draining into the chest can be managed successfully with open wound management and NGT drainage. Stenting and endoscopic vacuum-assisted closure systems are feasible, but not ideal in a high anastomosis due to positioning challenges and patient discomfort.

Anastomotic leaks in the chest are typically more challenging. Most patients will not decompensate clinically provided pleural drainage is adequate and mediastinitis is treated. If they are ignored, or intervention is delayed, the patient does not obtain "source control"; this can lead to worsening clinical condition and, frequently, a larger anastomotic leak, or even progression to gastric tip necrosis or fistula to the airway. Treatment options include conservative drainage and observation, nasogastric drainage, antibiotics, endoscopic stenting, endoscopic vacuum-assisted closure system, and surgical repair or re-anastomosis.

In the case of gastric tip necrosis, as in SISS Grade 4, choices include resection of the gastric tip and re-anastomosis in stable patients with limited contamination, or esophageal diversion with a cervical esophagostomy, also known as a "spit fistula." This complication is discussed later in this article.

In 2017, Liang and associates[14] published a large series of self-expanding esophageal stents, including 38 patients with anastomotic leak after esophagectomy. In this series, self-expanding fully covered or partially covered stents were used. Routine use of stent securing devices were used and the mean duration of stent use was 23 days. Thirteen patients (40%) required additional drainage procedures and 8 patients (23%) failed. Stent migration was lower in the partially covered stents when compared with the fully covered stent group. Another smaller study[15] included 19 patients with anastomotic leaks treated with stenting. In 5 patients (25%), closure of the leak failed and 4 went on to reoperation. Of these reoperations, 3 required resections and 1 required direct suture closure of the defect. In another study, Freeman and colleagues16,17 have been reporting results with stenting for more than a decade. In 2012, Freeman's group[16] published 187 esophageal leaks, which included perforations, anastomotic leaks, and fistulas. In that heterogenous population, only 15% of patients failed with esophageal stents and required traditional surgery. The investigators' results suggested that predictors of stent failure included proximal cervical leaks and anastomotic leaks associated with a more distal conduit leak. Malignancy or previous radiation therapy were not predictive of treatment failure. In another study, Freeman and colleagues[17] described successful healing in 17 patients with anastomotic leaks using stenting with 20% of patients requiring additional stenting. Few others have had the same level of success with esophageal stenting.

Although an important tool in management of anastomotic leaks, it is far from perfect. In addition to migration, need for re-stenting, exclusion of an inadequately drained mediastinum, and erosion into the aorta or airway must all be recognized as potential complications.

Endoscopic vacuum-assisted closure therapy (EVAC) uses traditional wound vacuum-assisted closure (VAC) principles to try to expedite closure of anastomotic leaks. EVAC is placed on an NGT (**Fig. 1**) at the level of an anastomosis or sometimes even through the anastomosis to drain, debride, and reapproximate the mediastinum

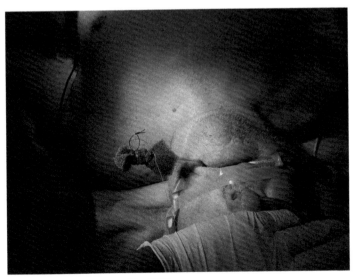

Fig. 1. Wound VAC sponge secured to NGT.

(Video 1). Although described more than a decade ago, few data exist, as demonstrated by a 2018 review article by Virgilio and colleagues,[18] which included only 209 patients reported in 29 papers. In one large retrospective study published after the review article, 20 patients with anastomotic leaks after esophagectomy were evaluated.[19] The mean defect was 1.75 cm. Success was accomplished in 19 (95%) of 20 patients over a median of 14.5 days and an average of 5 interventions. The authors also reported a trend for longer treatment in patients with larger anastomotic defects. Additional endoscopic reports of clipping, suturing, and using fibrin glue exist and may offer options in select cases but there is little compelling literature supporting these approaches.

Surgical reoperation can also be used. Repair of the prior anastomosis with additional suture and/or occlusion of the defect with a pedicle flap have all been described. On occasion, provided contamination is not excessive and the patient is stable, takedown of the anastomosis and re-anastomosis can be successful.

GASTRIC TIP NECROSIS

Gastric tip necrosis is fortunately a less common problem but associated with great morbidity. Occurring in approximately 1.5% of esophagectomies, it can be the result of technical issues that lead to impaired or damaged blood supply, or to patient malperfusion in sepsis or other low cardiac output states.

Strategies to avoid this complication include preservation of blood supply and optimizing perfusion postoperatively. Operative techniques to preserve blood supply include avoiding injury to the left gastroepiploic artery either by direct trauma or manipulation, or by early division before its termination on the greater curvature of the stomach. Preservation of the right gastric artery is another approach to maximize conduit blood supply. Another technique is creating a wider conduit, specifically avoiding too narrow a conduit. Maximizing postoperative perfusion includes focusing on cardiac output and maintaining a euvolemic state. Although there are no data to suggest a benefit of dopamine postoperatively, it has been used by many in the hopes of maximizing blood flow. Avoidance of vasopressors or, at least, judicious use of vasopressors to avoid constriction is likely of value.

PNEUMONIA/ASPIRATION EVENTS

Pneumonia and aspiration events occur more often than any other complication following esophagectomy, and the consequences can be devastating and can result in significant mortality.[6] In 2004, Law and colleagues[20] published a series of 421 patients in whom 55% of all mortalities were the consequence of pneumonia. Defining pneumonia has been a challenge and is variable throughout the literature. In our previous work, we used pulmonary infiltrate with positive cultures.[5] Frequently, pneumonia occurs because of other complications, such as aspiration following recurrent laryngeal nerve paralysis (RLNP), respiratory failure secondary to anastomotic leak, or reflux secondary to delayed gastric emptying. Because of the variable etiologies, a simple answer on how to avoid pneumonia in our patients evades us.

Treatment for pneumonia seems relatively simple, including antibiotic treatment of isolated bacteria, but in caring for such a patient the clinician must search for the cause and try to prevent it. When the pneumonia is a result of delayed gastric emptying, reintervention endoscopically or avoidance of per oral nutrition may be necessary until the patient's clinical status improves. Although mitigation of these and other factors is important, a firm understanding of how we can reduce the occurrence is important. Law demonstrated that increased age, tumors above the level of tracheal bifurcations, and prolonged operations were associated with an increased risk of pneumonia. In patients older than 70, the risk of developing pneumonia was twice as high, and the risk of mortality was fourfold. Our group looked at how surgical approaches influenced pulmonary complications.[21] In this multicenter trial, the data suggest that pulmonary complications were less frequent when thoracotomy was avoided and when patients were extubated immediately following surgery. We also demonstrated on multivariate analysis that pneumonia was more common with advancing age, and in the absence of a pyloric drainage procedure, and less common following MIE. This last point was supported by a recent meta-analysis of 1284 patients, and showed an overall reduction in the incidence of respiratory complications after MIE when compared with open techniques.[22]

Although some clinicians attempt to limit the risk of aspiration by limiting oral intake postoperatively this is contrary to many of the Enhanced Recovery after Surgery initiatives. Wang and colleagues[23] looked at patients with esophageal cancer to evaluate early enteral nutrition compared with later feeding more than 72 hours postoperatively. The early enteral feeding group had lower thoracic drainage, earlier first bowel movement, and shorter hospital stay than those who started enteral feeding after 72 hours. Furthermore, pneumonia was the highest in the late-feeding group. Mahmoodzadeh and colleagues[24] compared early oral feeding (EOF) on postoperative day 1 with delayed oral feeding in patients undergoing esophagectomy, and found that EOF alone was associated with shorter length of stay, fewer readmissions, and fewer complications.

VOCAL CORD PARALYSIS/RECURRENT LARYNGEAL NERVE PARALYSIS

Vocal cord paralysis occurs in 4.2% of patients undergoing esophagectomy as a result of injury to the recurrent laryngeal nerve.[6] Although more common with cervical anastomosis than intrathoracic anastomosis, it can occur in both; it is also more common in McKeown esophagectomy compared with transhiatal esophagectomy.[25] Vocal cord paralysis is associated with a longer length of stay and increased pulmonary complications. Nearly 50% of patients with RLNP after esophagectomy have respiratory complications.[26] Familiarity with cervical anatomy is critical to minimize this complication. Vocal cord paralysis should be suspected clinically if the patient has a hoarse voice, aspiration or cough with oral intake, or unexplained dyspnea due to loss of auto–positive end expiratory pressure. Evaluation is performed easily at the bedside with flexible laryngoscopy and does not require sedation.

The need for intervention is based on severity of symptoms. Studies show that half of patients with RLNP recover at 6 months without intervention.[25] In our practice, we are very aggressive regarding transoral vocal cord injection for medialization despite a paucity of data to support this approach. Friedman and colleagues[27] evaluated 32 patients undergoing early transoral injection of absorbable hyaluronic acid and 20 (68%) avoided any other intervention. Success in this series was defined by adequate voice and included both surgical and nonsurgical patients. Others have looked at improvement of swallowing with early intervention[28] and data here suggest that injection can markedly reduce the risk of aspiration and its sequala. Our ability to extrapolate directly to the post-esophagectomy patient is limited but clinical improvement for all symptoms can be dramatic and the procedure is low-risk.

CHYLOTHORAX

Chylothorax occurs approximately 5% of the time following esophagectomy.[6] It can range in severity, but the sequela includes decreased immunologic function, poor nutrition, and even death. Injury to the thoracic duct or its tributaries can occur due to direct transection, resection of tumor bed in the case of bulky tumor, or even from mass ligation. Gupta and colleagues[29] reported that risk factors include middle third tumors and difficult lymphadenectomy, irrespective of surgical approach. Others have attempted to prevent the occurrence by preemptive thoracic duct ligation at the time of the surgery. Jínek and colleagues[30] looked at routine thoracic duct ligation versus nonligation and found no reduction in the occurrence of chylothorax. Other groups have demonstrated reduced chylothorax with selective en-bloc ligation. Lin and colleagues[31] demonstrated reduced chylothorax with selective intraoperative thoracic duct ligation. The first group underwent mass ligation of the thoracic duct regardless of findings and the occurrence of chylothorax was 9.1%. In the second group, 9.5% demonstrated an intraoperative thoracic duct leak (with provocative use of 120 mL of olive oil) and underwent ligation. In the second group, undergoing selective ligation, none developed a postoperative chylothorax.

For those patients who do develop chylothorax postoperatively, treatment options include conservative management, embolization of the cisterna chyli, or surgical liga-tion. Attempted conservative management may be appropriate in patients who have low output or are less safe to endure another operation on a short-term basis. Frequently conservative management includes Octreotide 100 μg 3 times a day, restricted fat intake diet, pleural drainage, and occasionally pleurodesis. In 2018, Rei-senauer and colleagues[32] published a paper analyzing 97 iatrogenic (surgical) chylo-thoraces, of which 46 followed esophagectomy. The success rate for conservative management in the esophagectomy group was merely 32%. Patients with higher drainage were less likely to resolve without intervention. In this study, 40 patients un-derwent attempted embolization. Of those, the cisterna chyli could only be identified in 19 patients (48%) and was subsequently successful in 15 patients (38%). In the same publication, operative ligation was successful in 85% of patients. Although reopera-tion may not always succeed, most patients have good results. Brinkman and associ-ates[33] reported successful duct ligation in 15 of 15 post-esophagectomy chylothoraces. **Fig. 2** demonstrates 3 sequential steps and images associated with a successful embolization of post-esophagectomy chyle leak.

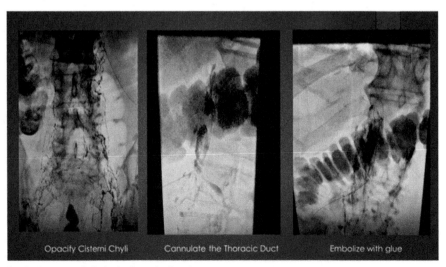

Fig. 2. Process of chyle leak embolization.

To summarize, post-esophagectomy chylothorax is not frequently resolved with conservative management. On occasion, a short trial for patients with low-output chylothorax may be reasonable but prolonged conservative management is an error in judgment. In patients who are stable and doing well, we advocate for expeditious reoperation via the right chest. For someone with recent prior thoracoscopy, this is a well-tolerated and highly successful approach and results in shortened recovery.[33] Cisterna chyli embolization is also a reasonable approach but not as successful as surgery. Embolization is successful in fewer than 40% of patients, which is fewer than half of patients who undergo surgery. In our practice, we use this approach for patients who are too fragile for surgery or who fail surgical ligation.

TRACHEOESOPHAGEAL FISTULA

Tracheoesophageal Fistula (TEF) may present as an acute or nonacute postoperative complication. Nonacute patients frequently present with recurrent pneumonia or coughing of food following oral intake. In this group, staple line erosion into airway or lung parenchyma occurs over time. Treatment is surgical, although stents may be temporizing. Surgical repair includes takedown of fistula and insertion of buttressing material between the closure. Acute TEF occurs from an anastomotic leak that is, not well controlled and/or allowed to fester, or after direct iatrogenic membranous airway injury during the primary operation. This injury can occur anywhere in the central airway but is particularly common in the left membranous airway due to operative angles. Most of these cases will present shortly after surgery with aspiration. Occasionally, routine postoperative esophagram can identify it or erroneously reporting it as an aspiration event. If an injury to the airway is identified intraoperatively, as shown in **Fig. 3**, we advocate for direct closure and coverage to separate the conduit/anastomosis from the airway. If the fistula is discovered postoperatively in days or weeks following surgery, it should be addressed in short order. Diagnosis is suspected

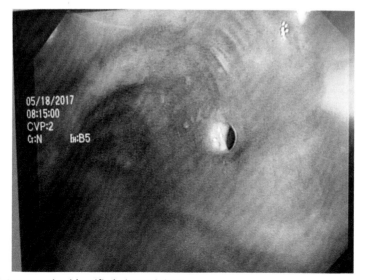

Fig. 3. Intraoperative identified airway injury.

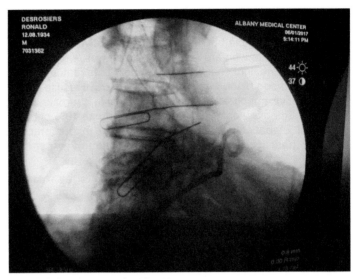

Fig. 4. Bronchial defect associated with TEF.

clinically and radiographically but confirmed via bronchoscopy as shown in **Fig. 4.** Although reports exist of successful management with airway and esophageal stenting,[34] failures are frequent but less commonly reported.[35] This approach appears to be only a temporizing measure in most cases. Stents can be placed across the airway or esophagus or both.[34] **Fig. 5** shows an airway stent being deployed in the left mainstem bronchus for a thermal injury during esophagectomy. Appropriate treatment includes reoperation with mobilization of the gastric conduit to gain access for repair

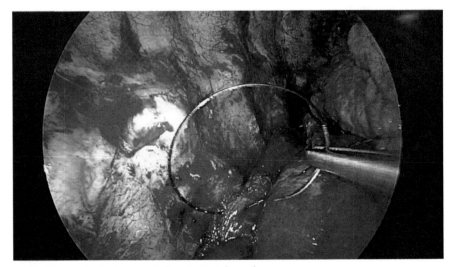

Fig. 5. Airway stent placed in left mainstem bronchus.

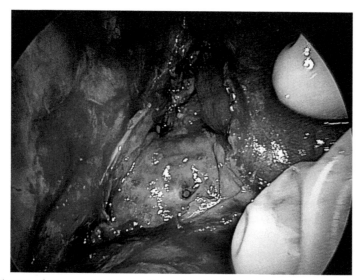

Fig. 6. Closure of airway with interposition of pedicled intercostal flap.

and buttress of airway as shown in **Fig. 6**. If a patient has a TEF associated with an anastomotic leak, the surgeon should consider diversion of esophagus or recreation of an anastomosis more proximally away from the airway repair.

DELAYED GASTRIC EMPTYING

Delayed gastric emptying is a complex issue and results from several confounding factors. This finding can be an immediate postoperative complication or a long-term condition. Frequently the clinician considers the status of the pylorus as being paramount and in some case it may be. In other cases, delayed gastric emptying is complex and interrelated between subjective complaints and objective interpretations of radiographic findings. Some people have argued that functionally, a narrow tube might be superior, but the data do not support this notion. Occasionally the conduit may be rotated or narrowed at the hiatus. In other cases, the conduit becomes distended and, with time, less functional. Occasionally, a post-esophagectomy hiatal hernia compresses the conduit extrinsically and repair results in resolution of symptoms. The clinician must consider all these issues to help the patient.

Pyloric drainage procedures have long been considered a priority following esophagectomy; denervation of the esophagus is considered a risk factor for delayed emptying. Urschel and colleagues[36] published a meta-analysis in 2002 demonstrating a reduced early complications due to delayed emptying when emptying procedures were performed. In 2009, we reported a prospective study demonstrating botulism toxin (Botox) injection of the pylorus during esophagectomy avoids delayed emptying in 96% of patients.[37] On the contrary in 2014, Eldaif and colleagues[38] reported increased reflux with no improvement in emptying with pyloric injection; they concluded that pyloromyotomy was superior to Botox injection and pyloroplasty during esophagectomy. For patients who develop postoperative emptying problems, reintervention with balloon dilation and Botox injection has been shown to improve symptoms in some patients.[37] This issue remains unsolved as a result of so many variables that interact in a wide range of patients to determine objective and subjective findings of dysphagia. Zhang and colleagues[39] looked at a large series of patients who received esophagectomies who did not undergo emptying procedures. Using univariate analysis, the only predictor of delayed gastric emptying was using a whole stomach as a gastric substitute. For patients with delayed gastric emptying problems, surgeons should exclude reversible issues like a hypertonic pylorus, a post-esophagectomy hernia, rotation of the conduit, and tumor recurrence. If one of these is found, the focus turns to intervention and even revision in some cases. In the absence of an anatomic abnormality, efforts should focus on prokinetic agents and dietary modifications although prokinetics are frequently ineffective.[40]

MORTALITY

The mortality following esophagectomy has been substantially reduced. In a multi-institutional Phase 2 study looking at MIE, mortality was 2.1%.[3] Although higher in the Society of Thoracic Surgeons database, there have been significant improvements in the past 20 years.

To maintain low mortality, a broad approach is important. Although a standard surgical approach, avoiding thoracotomy, for example, can help, it is only part of the answer. Patient selection is important as well as neoadjuvant treatment and nutritional status before surgery. Successful management of complications that occur in esophagectomy patients is critical to maximize survival and quality of life. Inappropriate or untimely treatment of anastomotic leaks, delayed emptying, chyle leaks, atrial fibrillation, and RLNP can all contribute to increased mortality.

To optimize results, the surgeon must have a firm understanding of the various complications, both common and uncommon, that can occur. The surgeon should be an expert endoscopist, as esophagoscopy is a critical component of evaluation, diagnosis, and management of many of the complications. In addition, the surgical team should focus on operative techniques and approaches that minimize the occurrence of complications and be ready, expeditious, and flexible in the management of them.

SUMMARY

Complications are common following esophagectomy regardless of the approach. The surgical team needs to be aware of complications, both frequent and infrequent, and how to manage them appropriately. Studies demonstrating or identifying novel or superior techniques that can be applied esophagectomy are of the utmost importance.

CLINICS CARE POINTS

- Grade 3 or 4 complications occur in 50% of esophagectomy patients.
- Familiarity of post esophagectomy complications is paramount to optimize outcomes.
- Both Technical complications and non-technical complications occur, and the surgeon should be prepared to manage both.

SUPPLEMENTARY DATA

Supplementary data to this article can be found online at https://doi.org/10.1016/j.suc.2021.03.013.

REFERENCES

1. He H, Chen N, Hou Y, et al. Trends in the incidence and survival of patients with esophageal cancer: a SEER database analysis. Thorac Cancer 2020;11(5): 1121–8.
2. Then EO, Lopez M, Saleem S, et al. Esophageal cancer: an updated surveillance epidemiology and end results database analysis. World J Oncol 2020;11(2): 55–64.
3. Luketich JD, Pennathur A, Franchetti Y, et al. Minimally invasive esophagectomy: results of a prospective phase II multicenter trial-the eastern cooperative oncology group (E2202) study. Ann Surg 2015;261(4):702–7.
4. Bizekis C, Kent MS, Luketich JD, et al. Initial experience with minimally invasive Ivor Lewis esophagectomy. Ann Thorac Surg 2006;82(2):402–6 [discussion: 406–7].
5. Fabian T, Martin JT, McKelvey AA, et al. Minimally invasive esophagectomy: a teaching hospital's first year experience. Dis Esophagus 2008;21(3):220–5.
6. Low DE, Alderson D, Ceccpnello I, et al. International consensus on standardization of data collection for complications associated with esophagectomy: Esophagectomy Complications Consensus Group (ECCG). Ann Surg 2015;262(2): 286–94.
7. Low DE, Kuppusamy MK, Alderson D, et al. Benchmarking complications associated with esophagectomy. Ann Surg 2019;269(2):291–8.
8. Ozawa S, Koyanagi K, Ninomiya Y, et al. Postoperative complications of minimally invasive esophagectomy for esophageal cancer. Ann Gastroenterol Surg 2020; 4(2):126–34.
9. Scarpa M, Valente S, Alfieri R, et al. Systematic review of health-related quality of life after esophagectomy for esophageal cancer. World J Gastroenterol 2011; 17(42):4660–74.
10. Cooper JS, Guo M, Herskovic A, et al. Chemoradiotherapy of locally advanced esophageal cancer long-term follow-up of a prospective randomized trial (RTOG 85-01). JAMA 1999;281(17):1623–7.
11. Dubecz A, Sepesi B, Salvador R, et al. Surgical resection for locoregional esophageal cancer is underutilized in the United States. J Am Coll Surg 2010;211(6): 754–61.
12. Peel AL, Taylor EW. Proposed definitions for the audit of postoperative infection: a discussion paper. Surgical Infection Study Group. Ann R Coll Surg Engl 1991; 73(6):385–8.
13. Verstegen MHP, Bouwense SAW, Workum FV, et al. Management of intrathoracic and cervical anastomotic leakage after esophagectomy for esophageal cancer: a systematic review. World J Emerg Surg 2019;14:17.
14. Liang DH, Hwang E, Meisenbach LM, et al. Clinical outcomes following self-expanding metal stent placement for esophageal salvage. J Thorac Cardiovasc Surg 2017;154(3):1145–50.
15. Tuebergen D, Rijcken E, Mennigen R, et al. Treatment of thoracic esophageal anastomotic leaks and esophageal perforations with endoluminal stents: efficacy and current limitations. J Gastrointest Surg 2008;12(7):1168–76.
16. Freeman RK, Ascioti AJ, Giannini T, et al. Analysis of unsuccessful esophageal stent placements for esophageal perforation, fistula, or anastomotic leak. Ann Thorac Surg 2012;94(3):959–64 [discussion: 964–5].

17. Freeman RK, Vyverberg A, Ascioti AJ. Esophageal stent placement for the treatment of acute intrathoracic anastomotic leak after esophagectomy. Ann Thorac Surg 2011;92(1):204–8 [discussion: 208].
18. Virgilio E, Ceci D, Cavallini M. Surgical Endoscopic Vacuum-assisted Closure Therapy (EVAC) in treating anastomotic leakages after major resective surgery of esophageal and gastric cancer. Anticancer Res 2018;38(10):5581–7.
19. Min YW, Kim T, Lee H, et al. Endoscopic vacuum therapy for postoperative esophageal leak. BMC Surg 2019;19(1):37.
20. Law S, Wong KH, Kwok KF, et al. Predictive factors for postoperative pulmonary complications and mortality after esophagectomy for cancer. Ann Surg 2004; 240(5):791–800.
21. Bakhos CT, Fabian T, Oyasiji TO, et al. Impact of the surgical technique on pulmonary morbidity after esophagectomy. Ann Thorac Surg 2012;93(1):221–6 [discussion: 226–7].
22. Nagpal K, Ahmed K, Vats A, et al. Is minimally invasive surgery beneficial in the management of esophageal cancer? A meta-analysis. Surg Endosc 2010;24(7): 1621–9.
23. Wang G, Chen H, Liu J, et al. A comparison of postoperative early enteral nutrition with delayed enteral nutrition in patients with esophageal cancer. Nutrients 2015; 7(6):4308–17.
24. Mahmoodzadeh H, Shoar S, Sirati F, et al. Early initiation of oral feeding following upper gastrointestinal tumor surgery: a randomized controlled trial. Surg Today 2015;45(2):203–8.
25. Scholtemeijer MG, Seesing MFJ, Benkman HJF, et al. Recurrent laryngeal nerve injury after esophagectomy for esophageal cancer: incidence, management, and impact on short- and long-term outcomes. J Thorac Dis 2017;9(Suppl 8): S868–78.
26. Gockel I, Kneist W, Keilmann A, et al. Recurrent laryngeal nerve paralysis (RLNP) following esophagectomy for carcinoma. Eur J Surg Oncol 2005;31(3):277–81.
27. Friedman AD, Burns JA, Heaton JT, et al. Early versus late injection medialization for unilateral vocal cord paralysis. Laryngoscope 2010;120(10):2042–6.
28. Zuniga S, Ebersole B, Jamal N. Improved swallow outcomes after injection laryngoplasty in unilateral vocal fold immobility. Ear Nose Throat J 2018;97(8): 250–6.
29. Gupta R, Singh H, Kalia S, et al. Chylothorax after esophagectomy for esophageal cancer: risk factors and management. Indian J Gastroenterol 2015;34(3): 240–4.
30. Jínek T, Adamčík L, Duda M, et al. Prophylactic ligation of the thoracic duct in the prevention of chylothorax after esophagectomy. Rozhl Chir 2018;97(7):328–34.
31. Lin Y, Li Z, Li G, et al. Selective en masse ligation of the thoracic duct to prevent chyle leak after esophagectomy. Ann Thorac Surg 2017;103(6):1802–7.
32. Reisenauer JS, Puig CA, Reisenauer CJ, et al. Treatment of postsurgical chylothorax. Ann Thorac Surg 2018;105(1):254–62.
33. Brinkmann S, Schroeder W, Junggeburth K, et al. Incidence and management of chylothorax after Ivor Lewis esophagectomy for cancer of the esophagus. J Thorac Cardiovasc Surg 2016;151(5):1398–404.
34. Schweigert M, Dubecz A, Beron M, et al. Management of anastomotic leakage-induced tracheobronchial fistula following oesophagectomy: the role of endoscopic stent insertion. Eur J Cardiothorac Surg 2012;41(5):e74–80.
35. Zisis C, Guillin A, Heyries L, et al. Stent placement in the management of oesophageal leaks. Eur J Cardiothorac Surg 2008;33(3):451–6.

36. Urschel JD, Blewett CJ, Young JEM, et al. Pyloric drainage (pyloroplasty) or no drainage in gastric reconstruction after esophagectomy: a meta-analysis of randomized controlled trials. Dig Surg 2002;19(3):160–4.
37. Martin JT, Federico JA, McKelvey AA, et al. Prevention of delayed gastric emptying after esophagectomy: a single center's experience with botulinum toxin. Ann Thorac Surg 2009;87(6):1708–13 [discussion: 1713–4].
38. Eldaif SM, Lee R, Adams KN, et al. Intrapyloric botulinum injection increases postoperative esophagectomy complications. Ann Thorac Surg 2014;97(6): 1959–64 [discussion: 1964–5].
39. Zhang L, Hou SC, Miao JB, et al. Risk factors for delayed gastric emptying in patients undergoing esophagectomy without pyloric drainage. J Surg Res 2017; 213:46–50.
40. Simpson PJ, Ooi C, Chong J, et al. Does the use of nizatidine, as a pro-kinetic agent, improve gastric emptying in patients post-oesophagectomy? J Gastrointest Surg 2009;13(3):432–7.

Moving?

Make sure your subscription moves with you!

To notify us of your new address, find your **Clinics Account Number** (located on your mailing label above your name), and contact customer service at:

Email: journalscustomerservice-usa@elsevier.com

800-654-2452 (subscribers in the U.S. & Canada)
314-447-8871 (subscribers outside of the U.S. & Canada)

Fax number: 314-447-8029

Elsevier Health Sciences Division
Subscription Customer Service
3251 Riverport Lane
Maryland Heights, MO 63043

*To ensure uninterrupted delivery of your subscription, please notify us at least 4 weeks in advance of move.

ELSEVIER

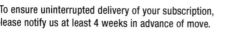

Printed and bound by CPI Group (UK) Ltd, Croydon, CR0 4YY

03/10/2024

01040400-0015